Difficult Cases in Primary Care: Paediatrics

SAMAR RAZAQ

MBChB, MRCGP, DRCOG, DCH, DGM

General Practitioner
Buckinghamshire

Radcliffe Publishing
London • New York

Radcliffe Publishing Ltd
St Mark's House
Shepherdess Walk
London N1 7BQ
United Kingdom

www.radcliffehealth.com

_____

British Library Cataloguing in Publication Data

A catalogue record for this book is available from the British Library.

ISBN-13: 978 184619 985 1

Typeset by Beautiful Words, Auckland, New Zealand
Printed and bound by Cadmus Communications, USA

Contents

Preface

This book is the second in the Difficult Cases in Primary Care series and aims to cover difficult scenarios that may be encountered in primary care. I find paediatrics to be a somewhat misleading term, as if it encompasses a definitive subset of patients who present with a particular set of conditions, all to be managed in a similar fashion. The 2-day-old newborn with jaundice represents a completely different diagnostic dilemma to the 16-year-old presenting with jaundice. No other specialty has to deal with such rapidly changing physiology and, hence, changing probabilities of differential diagnoses. General practitioners are required to maintain a breadth of knowledge covering the whole age group encompassing the specialty. In many cases the diagnosis may not be made in the general practitioner's surgery, but that is where the suspicion is often raised.

This book follows the format of the first book in the series. A case scenario is presented, followed by a detailed explanation of the condition and its management. This format is useful, as it presents the condition in a way that is likely to be encountered in real life. Modern exams also favour this format, as it mimics the objective structured clinical exams that many candidates have to undertake. The detailed explanation is then followed by questions for examination practice. The answers, along with a comprehensive explanation, are found at the end of the book. My hope is that paediatric and general practice examination candidates will find this an invaluable aid to their examination preparation.

Samar Razaq
March 2014

About the author

Dr Samar Razaq works as a general practitioner in Buckinghamshire. He graduated from the University of Birmingham in 2005. During his general practice training he completed diplomas in child health, geriatric medicine, and obstetrics and gynaecology. He is the author of this Difficult Cases in Primary Care series of books. Radcliffe published the first book in the series, *Difficult Cases in Primary Care: Women's Health*, in 2012. He currently resides in Buckinghamshire with his wife and three children.

List of abbreviations

ADHD	attention deficit hyperactivity disorder
ASD	autistic spectrum disorder
CAH	congenital adrenal hyperplasia
CF	cystic fibrosis
CFTR	cystic fibrosis transmembrane conductance regulator
CPK	creatine phosphokinase
CRP	C-reactive protein
DKA	diabetic ketoacidosis
DMD	Duchenne's muscular dystrophy
DMSA	dimercaptosuccinic acid
DSM-IV	*Diagnostic and Statistical Manual of Mental Disorders* (4th edition)
EEG	electroencephalogram
ENT	ear, nose and throat
ESR	erythrocyte sedimentation rate
FBC	full blood count
FS	febrile seizure
FTU	fingertip unit
GERD	gastro-oesophageal reflux disease
GP	general practitioner
HKD	hyperkinetic disorder
HSP	Henoch–Schönlein purpura
IBS	irritable bowel syndrome

ICD-10	*International Statistical Classification of Diseases and Related Health Problems* (10th edition)
IEM	inborn error of metabolism
IgA	immunoglobulin A
IgA1	immunoglobulin A1
IgE	immunoglobulin E
IgG	immunoglobulin G
IgM	immunoglobulin M
IVIG	intravenous immunoglobulin
JIA	juvenile idiopathic arthritis
MCUG	micturating cystourethrogram
MPH	mid-parental height
NICE	National Institute for Health and Care Excellence
o/e	on examination
OOH	out-of-hours
PPI	proton pump inhibitor
RAP	recurrent abdominal pain
RF	rheumatoid factor
RSV	respiratory syncytial virus
SIDS	sudden infant death syndrome
T1DM	type 1 diabetes mellitus
T2DM	type 2 diabetes mellitus
UK	United Kingdom
USS	ultrasound scan
UTI	urinary tract infection
VSD	ventricular septal defect
VUR	vesicoureteric reflux

Febrile seizures

You see 15-month-old John in clinic with a 24-hour history of fever, runny nose and tugging at the right ear. On examination, the child appears well and is afebrile. You note that the right tympanic membrane is bulging, with an inflamed appearance. You make a diagnosis of otitis media and send mum home with a prescription of amoxicillin. Two days later mum, who is an orthopaedic nurse, returns with discharge papers from the paediatric ward. Later at night after you saw him, John developed a very high temperature of 39°C. As he lay in his cot, he suddenly started jerking. Mum says he appeared to go very stiff and he became unresponsive, with his eyes rolled upwards. Thinking that he was dying, mum dialled for the ambulance. By the time the ambulance crew arrived, the jerking had settled. John, however, remained semi-conscious and it was not until an hour later in the emergency department that he was completely back to normal. The paediatric discharge notes inform you that a lumbar puncture was performed. It, along with blood results, was normal. The final diagnosis was that of a simple febrile seizure (FS). Mum would like John to be referred for an electroencephalogram (EEG). She also enquires about prophylactic diazepam to stop seizures from occurring in the future.

Which of the following statements is/are *true*?

a   A lumbar puncture is always indicated when a child presents with a FS.
b   It is good practice to perform blood tests to get an idea regarding the severity of the infection.
c   An EEG should have been carried out during the admission, as it is a most sensitive test when carried out within 24 hours of the seizure.
d   Long-term outcome after a FS is excellent in terms of intellectual capability and behaviour.
e   There is strong and convincing evidence that FSs cause damage to the hippocampus, resulting in an increased risk of developing temporal lobe epilepsy.

Answer: d

FSs are a commonly encountered paediatric problem occurring in 2%–5% of all children. There are slight variations in how a FS may be defined; however, it is commonly described as a seizure associated with fever in the absence of underlying intracranial infection or any other recognised cause of seizure activity such as trauma, epilepsy or electrolyte imbalance. FSs are more common in children between the ages of 6 months and 3 years, with a peak incidence at the age of 18 months. Onset after the age of 6 is uncommon. A fever of greater that 38°C is usually quoted as being required to make the diagnosis of a FS. Despite this, the fever may not be the cause of the FS. This is backed by studies showing that the use of antipyretics is not effective in preventing the recurrence of FSs. A randomised, double-blind, placebo-controlled trial performed by van Stuijvenberg and colleagues (1998) randomised 230 children between the ages of 1 and 4 to receive either ibuprofen or placebo regularly during a febrile episode until adequate temperature control had been achieved. These children had had a FS in the past and were deemed at high risk of having a recurrence. Analysis at the end of the study did not show any difference in the risk of recurrent FSs. Other studies have yielded similar results with paracetamol. It is possible that endogenous proteins such as interleukin 1, released during a pyretic episode, increase neuronal excitability and lower the seizure threshold, thus linking the fever with the seizure. The exact mechanism, however, remains elusive.

The strongest risk factor for having a FS is a history of FSs in a first-degree relative. For most children this will be a solitary event; however, a FS will recur in approximately a third of children. They are at the highest risk within the first year of the initial event. FSs may be classified as simple and complex. Simple seizures, which make up the large majority of FSs, are short in duration (lasting shorter than 10 minutes), have generalised tonic–clonic seizure activity, resolve spontaneously and do not recur within 24 hours. Seizures are classified as complex if they last for longer than 15 minutes, have focal seizure activity or reoccur within 24 hours. Febrile status epilepticus is a form of complex FS in which the seizure lasts for more than 30 minutes. The differentiation is important, as a complex FS is associated with an increased risk of developing epilepsy when compared with a simple FS (if all three features are present, the risk of developing epilepsy is approximately 50%). Other factors increasing the risk of developing epilepsy include a family history of epilepsy and neurological abnormalities. Interestingly, fever duration of less than 1 hour prior to seizure onset is also associated with an increased risk of developing epilepsy later in life. In contrast, a simple FS with none of the aforementioned factors is associated with a 2.4% risk of developing epilepsy (a modest rise above the 1.4% risk for the background population). Parents should be reassured that long-term prognosis in terms of intellect, academic achievement, memory and behaviour is good.

The first step in the management is to confirm the diagnosis. As is the case in the scenario given earlier, it is not uncommon for seizure activity to have terminated by the time the child reaches the emergency department. As with all cases, a good history is vital. Alternative diagnoses, including rigors, syncope, reflex anoxic seizures, febrile delirium and breath-holding attacks, should be considered. The age of the child and degree of illness will further determine how the child is managed, once the diagnosis of a FS is made. The first step would be to determine the source of infection. If this can be accurately determined, further investigations may not be indicated. Examination of the ear, throat, chest and nervous system is mandatory. A urine dip should be performed to rule out a urinary tract infection. A FS is not an indication for routine blood tests and they should only be performed if a specific indication exists. A decision needs to be made whether a lumbar puncture is indicated and this will be determined by the suspected source of infection. If meningitis or encephalitis is suspected, a lumbar puncture should be performed unless contraindicated. In the older child (above 2 years of age), the clinical diagnosis of meningeal irritation may be easier to make. In the absence of suggestive signs (such as neck stiffness, photophobia), with a clear alternative source of infection, a lumbar puncture, therefore, would not be necessary. However, in the younger child – particularly, a child younger than 1 year of age – the diagnosis may be difficult on clinical grounds because of the subtlety with which the child may present. Poor feeding, irritability and lethargy may be signs of meningitis and in such a scenario a lumbar puncture should be strongly considered. There is no evidence that EEG, done at the time of presentation or up to a month later, has any prognostic or diagnostic benefit. This is the case for simple and complex FSs, and it should therefore not be routinely performed. A FS may herald the onset of an epileptic disorder, such as Dravet's syndrome, in which case an EEG will be performed. However, the suspicion of such syndromes is raised after a single or multiple FS. In the absence of abnormal neurological findings, there is no need for neuroimaging for either simple or complex FSs. In the presence of neurological abnormalities, non-urgent magnetic resonance imaging should be organised.

Immediate management to terminate the seizure is indicated if the seizure is prolonged. Treatment should be given if the seizure lasts longer than 5 minutes. Rectal diazepam or buccal midazolam at a dose of 0.5 mg/kg is effective at terminating seizures. Midazolam may also be given intranasally. They are the drugs of choice in the primary care setting because of the likelihood of not having intravenous access. In a study comparing the two benzodiazepines in children aged 6 months and older attending hospital, buccal midazolam was found to be more effective than rectal diazepam in terminating the seizure within 10 minutes for at least an hour (McIntyre, et al., 2005). If the seizure is not terminated within 10 minutes of delivery of the drug or the seizure recurs, then an ambulance should be called to organise hospital admission. Long-term management is centred on parent reassurance and explanation of the condition.

The mother in this case enquires about prophylaxis. As discussed earlier, evidence in favour of regular antipyretic prescribing to prevent the recurrence of a FS is lacking. Nevertheless, antipyretics should be used to make the child more comfortable. Long-term anticonvulsant treatment has been used in the past but is no longer recommended, because of the lack of evidence of its effectiveness in reducing the risk of a recurrence or reducing the risk of epilepsy. Coupled with an unfavourable side effect profile, it is not usually difficult to convince parents against the use of regular anti-epileptic medication. Since the use of regular preventive medication has fallen out of use, intermittent use of preventive benzodiazepines has gained some favour. Studies have shown intermittent use of diazepam, during a febrile episode, to be effective in preventing a recurrence of FS. Side effects found to be associated with diazepam use in such a manner included lethargy, irritability and ataxia, with up to a third of children affected in one study. A discussion with the parent should revolve around whether preventing a recurrence is necessary or not. Risk factors for an increased risk of recurrence include first FS below the age of 18 months, history of FSs in a first-degree relative, shorter duration of fever (<1 hour) prior to seizure onset, seizure occurring at relatively lower temperature (35% within 1 year with a recorded temperature of 38.3°C, reducing to 13% with a temperature of 40.6°C or higher) and multiple seizures occurring in the same febrile episode. In the absence of these features, parents may wish not to embark on benzodiazepine prophylaxis.

Examination practice: funny turns

Options for questions 1–3:

a West's syndrome

b breath-holding attacks

c Sandifer's syndrome

d absence seizures

e benign rolandic epilepsy

f Angelman's syndrome

g pavor nocturnus

h panic attacks.

Questions 1–3 are about children presenting with a 'funny turn'. From the list of options provided, choose the most appropriate diagnosis that fits the clinical presentation. Each option may be used once, more than once or not at all.

1 A 5-year-old girl is seen in the epilepsy clinic. She is noted to have coarse features. Mum tells you that she has sudden outbursts of unprovoked laughter and is fascinated by running water.

2 An 8-year-old boy presents with tingling in his mouth, lips and gums on waking in the morning. On a few occasions dad has noticed his speech to be unclear.

3 A 2-year-old boy passes out after he is told off. Mum says that he was crying and became red in the face prior to passing out. She does not report any abnormal jerking and he regained consciousness within a minute.

4 Which of the following statements regarding retinoblastoma are *true*?
   a Retinoblastoma is the commonest primary ocular tumour in children.
   b Retinoblastoma is a life-threatening condition, with an approximately 50% mortality rate in the first year in the UK.
   c The diagnosis of retinoblastoma is delayed in most cases.
   d A new-onset strabismus may be a sign of a retinoblastoma.
   e Children with an inherited form of retinoblastoma are at an increased risk of developing non-ocular cancers later in life.

5 Which of the following signs is usually positive in Marfan's syndrome?
   a Steinberg's sign

   b Gower's sign

   c Rovsing's sign

   d Scarf sign

   e Murphy's sign

Bibliography

American Academy of Pediatrics, Provisional Committee on Quality Improvement, Subcommittee on Febrile Seizures. Practice parameter: the neurodiagnostic evaluation of the child with a first simple febrile seizure. *Pediatrics*. 1996 May; **97**(5): 769–72; discussion 773–5.

Barr DGD, Crofton PM, Goel KM. Disorders of bone, joints and connective tissue. In: Campbell AGM, McIntosh N, editors. *Forfar and Arneil's Textbook of Pediatrics*. 5th ed. New York, NY: Churchill Livingstone; 1998. pp. 1544–615.

Berg AT, Shinnar S, Hauser WA, *et al.* A prospective study of recurrent febrile seizures. *N Engl J Med*. 1992 Oct 15; **327**(16): 1122–7.

Brown JK, Minns RA. Disorders of the central nervous system: surgical paediatrics. In: Campbell AGM, McIntosh N, editors. *Forfar and Arneil's Textbook of Pediatrics*. 5th ed. New York, NY: Churchill Livingstone; 1998. pp. 641–846.

Butros LJ, Abramson DH, Dunkel IJ. Delayed diagnosis of retinoblastoma: analysis of degree, cause, and potential consequences. *Pediatrics*. 2002 Mar; **109**(3): E45.

Childhood Eye Cancer Trust. *Campaign Launched after 72% of Children had Eye Cancer Treatment Delayed by GPs*. London: Childhood Eye Cancer Trust; 13 May 2013. Available at: www.chect.org.uk/cms/images/PDFs/rb%20week%202013%20final.pdf (accessed 10 October 2013).

Cuestas E. Is routine EEG helpful in the management of complex febrile seizures? *Arch Dis Child*. 2004 Mar; **89**(3): 290.

El-Radhi AS, Barry W. Do antipyretics prevent febrile convulsions? *Arch Dis Child*. 2003 Jul; **88**(7): 641–2.

Epilepsy Action. *Angelman Syndrome*. Leeds: Epilepsy Action; updated March 2012. Available at: www.epilepsy.org.uk/info/syndromes/angelman-syndrome (accessed 12 January 2013).

Halford L, Cole T, Kingston J, *et al.* Retinoblastoma for life. *Focus: The Royal College of Ophthalmologists*. 2008; Summer: 5–6.

Joint Working Group of the Research Unit of the Royal College of Physicians and the British Paediatric Association. Guidelines for the management of convulsions with fever. *BMJ.* 1991 Sep 14; **303**(6803): 634–6.

McIntyre J, Robertson S, Norris E, *et al.* Safety and efficacy of buccal midazolam versus rectal diazepam for emergency treatment of seizures in children: a randomised controlled trial. *Lancet.* 2005 Jul 16–22; **366**(9481): 205–10.

Rosman NP, Colton T, Labazzo J, *et al.* A controlled trial of diazepam administered during febrile illnesses to prevent recurrence of febrile seizures. *N Engl J Med.* 1993 Jul 8; **329**(2): 79–84.

Sadleir LG, Scheffer IE. Febrile seizures. *BMJ.* 2007 Feb 10; **334**(7588): 307–11.

Srinivasan J, Wallace KA, Scheffer IE. Febrile seizures. *Aust Fam Physician.* 2005 Dec; **34**(12): 1021–5.

Van Stuijvenberg M, Derksen-Lubsen G, Steyerberg EW, *et al.* Randomized, controlled trial of ibuprofen syrup administered during febrile illnesses to prevent febrile seizure recurrences. *Pediatrics.* 1998 Nov; **102**(5): e51. Available at: http://pediatrics.aappublications.org/content/102/5/e51.full.pdf+html (accessed 13 January 2013).

Waruiru C, Appleton R. Febrile seizures: an update. *Arch Dis Child.* 2004 Aug; **89**(8): 751–6.

Chronic constipation

Five-year-old Mark visits the surgery with mum. You note that he has been in and out of the surgery over the last year with problems related to constipation and faecal soiling. A whole host of laxatives have been prescribed at the different visits. Mum tells you that he was fully toilet-trained at the age of 3. He started to suffer from mild bouts of constipation when he joined nursery about a year ago. As time progressed the constipation seemed to worsen. Mark occasionally stands in the corner and crosses his legs, with his buttocks clenched, in obvious distress. Now mum increasingly finds loose stool on Mark's underwear, which he seems to be oblivious of passing. Over the last year mum would use laxatives for a few days but would have to stop within days, as diarrhoea would develop. Needless to say this is causing a huge amount of distress in the family and is also affecting Mark's self-esteem. He now seems reluctant to attend school and actively avoids attending the toilet, despite encouragement and promise of rewards. On further questioning you find that Mark was a term baby, passed meconium stool within 24 hours of birth and has been growing normally along the 50th centile. Examination reveals a slightly distended abdomen with palpable stool in the left lower quadrant. Mum is confused why every doctor she sees keeps prescribing laxatives when Mark seems to be constantly leaking loose stool.

Which of the following statements is/are *true*?

a Mark's symptoms are typical of chronic non-specific diarrhoea, otherwise known as toddler diarrhoea.

b Hirschsprung's disease is a common diagnosis in this age group.

c Encopresis (chronic faecal soiling at the age of 4 years and older) and constipation are closely linked with bladder dysfunction.

d Abdominal radiographs should be routinely performed in the evaluation of a child with constipation.

e Macrogol (polyethylene glycol) laxatives may be used if faecal impaction is suspected in the child.

Answer: c and e

Chronic constipation is a common but somewhat unglamorous paediatric problem. Understanding the underlying processes leading to constipation and its effective management are vital for primary care physicians. It is important to differentiate between functional and organic causes of constipation. Mark's case is that of functional constipation. Organic causes of constipation will be dealt with further in the questions following this particular case.

The prevalence of constipation is determined by the criteria used to define it. Constipation is present when the passage of stool is associated with either pain or difficulty (or both). The estimated prevalence is around 5%–30% in childhood. In a proportion of these children the problem will become chronic, which is associated with considerable physical, psychological and social morbidity. The underlying cause of idiopathic constipation is unclear. There is a possibility, as a child reaches toilet-training age, the stool is more prone to dryness, becomes harder and has longer transit times. However, it is not uncommon in clinical practice to see children where the chronic problem starts after an initial bout of constipation. This could have been caused by dehydration (for whatever reason), a stressful life event, medication causing constipation or a stressful toilet-training regimen at home or school. Matters are made worse, in some circumstances, when the family or the physician ignore the initial symptoms. The development of constipation results in bouts of abdominal pain and possible development of anal fissures. The child begins to associate the passage of stool with pain and hence actively avoids passing stool. Stool holding (manifested by standing in corners with legs crossed, buttocks clenched or rocking) and toilet refusal are manifestations of this active avoidance. This results in hardening of the stool in the rectum, making it more difficult to pass. The resulting expansion of the rectum and sigmoid colon makes them insensitive. The child stops feeling the normal contractions of the bowel, reducing his or her urge to defecate. This further hardens and enlarges the faecal mass in the distal bowel, leading to worsening constipation. A vicious cycle is thus set up that constantly propagates further constipation. Laxative use at this stage may result in looser stool 'bypassing' the hard faecal mass and causing troublesome soiling. Parents may mistake this overflow incontinence as resolution of the problem and prematurely stop the use of laxatives. Seeing different physicians at each visit to the surgery may exacerbate the issue, as only short-term fixes are offered with a dizzying array of laxatives. The importance of explaining the process to the parents (and child if possible) cannot be underestimated. Diagrams to show faecal impaction, rectal enlargement and insensitivity and overflow incontinence may be used to help parents understand what is happening and comprehend the rationale of the various treatment modalities. It also liberates the child from the stigma of the encopresis being a manifestation of a behavioural disorder.

Mark will need laxatives to help overcome his problem. However, it is worth mentioning a few other important management strategies, as maintenance of normal bowel movement after successful treatment will depend on important lifestyle changes. Stool holding can often be mistaken for straining by parents and caregivers. Explanation that fear of pain forces the child to contract the anal sphincter, thereby preventing passage of the faecal mass, may help in better management of the problem. The child should be encouraged to sit on the toilet daily. Fluid and fibre intake should be increased. One double-blind, randomised, placebo-controlled study (Loening-Baucke, *et al.*, 2004) found fibre (glucomannan) intake to be beneficial in the treatment of chronic constipation; success was determined by an increase in bowel movements, reduction in encopresis and reduction in abdominal pain. Another study observed that the increased intake of raw bran and high-fibre foods coupled with restrictions in dairy and other possible constipating foods also improved constipation in children. Cow's milk has been implicated in the cause of constipation in other studies too. One study (Iacono, *et al.*, 1995) followed 27 infants, initially on an unrestricted diet followed by a diet free of cow's milk protein. Twenty-one of the 27 infants showed symptom resolution, and 15 of those 21 infants demonstrated raised serum markers such as IgE and IgG, suggesting an allergic pathogenesis. A double-blind crossover study by the same authors further strengthened the link between cow's milk protein and constipation. Children who responded to a diet free of cow's milk protein were more likely to have inflammatory changes evident on rectal biopsy. It is, therefore, worthwhile suggesting a short period of a milk-free diet to see if this helps with symptoms. If the child responds to a milk-free diet, it is unclear when milk should be reintroduced into the diet. A small study, based on 18 infants (El-Hodhod, *et al.*, 2009), found that reintroducing milk after 12 months was associated with better tolerance to cow's milk protein after the reintroduction. Withdrawing milk from the diet for a year, however, may not be feasible for every child. Sorbitol-containing fruit juices (apple, pear) may be recommended in infants to help soften the stool.

The purpose of laxative therapy is to maintain a regular bowel habit. Parents should be made aware that treatment is likely to continue for some time beyond the achievement of a regular bowel movement because of the high risk of recurrence of constipation. Mark seems to be impacted. Impaction refers to the presence of a faecal mass palpable transabdominally or upon rectal examination. As this impacted mass is unlikely to pass on demand, it is imperative that disimpaction takes place prior to starting laxative therapy. If maintenance laxative treatment is started before disimpaction, there is a risk of increased faecal soiling as a result of overflow diarrhoea, as looser stool bypasses the impacted mass. There is no consensus on the best method of disimpaction but various agents have been used with reasonable success. Enemas, oral laxatives or suppositories may be used to promote disimpaction. One prospective, randomised controlled study (Bekkali, *et al.*, 2009) compared enemas with high-dose oral macrogols (polyethylene glycol) for the treatment of rectal faecal impaction and found both to be equally effective. Since enemas or suppositories may distress the child, a reasonable option would be to start disimpaction with oral macrogols. A systematic review by Candy and Belsey (2008) of the studies looking at the use of macrogol in children with constipation and faecal impaction concluded that it was an effective and well-tolerated first-line option. A reasonable regimen in this child, for disimpaction, would be to start with four sachets daily, gradually increasing to 12 sachets a day if needed. This can be used in combination with lactulose (another osmotic laxative) or stimulant laxatives such as senna, sodium picosulphate, bisacodyl or glycerol suppositories. If this does not work then an arachis oil enema (in those over 3 years of age) can be used as a faecal softener and lubricator. Sodium citrate or phosphate enemas may be used if disimpaction is not achieved by the methods mentioned. Occasionally, in constipation resistant to treatment, bowel cleansing preparations or manual evacuation under anaesthetic is needed under specialist supervision.

Once disimpaction has been achieved and maintenance therapy started with one or a combination of the laxatives mentioned here, regular review of the child is necessary. This is important to ensure that regular bowel movements have been established and that constipation is not reoccurring, and to answer any concerns the parents may have.

Examination practice: organic constipation

Options for questions 6–8:

a   cystic fibrosis

b   congenital anal stenosis

c   Hirschsprung's disease

d   hypothyroidism

e   spina bifida

f   neurofibromatosis

g   lead poisoning

h   spinal cord trauma

i   meconium plug syndrome

j   pyloric stenosis.

This is a non-exhaustive list of conditions that need to be considered in a child presenting with constipation. Questions 6–8 refer to children presenting with constipation. Choose the most likely diagnosis from the options provided.

6   A 6-year-old boy presents with chronic constipation. You are aware that he is also under the care of the child mental health team for antisocial behaviour, aggression and a low intelligence quotient. Mum seeks advice on how to deal with the constipation. She also asks how she can stop him from eating peeling paint and soil.

7   A 5-month-old girl presents to the surgery with mum. She is part of an Afghan refugee family who have moved to the country 2 months ago. The child was born at term, at home, with no complications. Mum tells you that her stool has always been small in size and little in quantity, much like toothpaste. More recently she has started to leak stool pretty much constantly. Examination reveals no stigmata of neurological disease.

8   A 2-day-old child presents with abdominal distension, reluctance to feed and bile-stained vomiting. A careful history reveals the child is yet to pass meconium. Rectal biopsy confirms the absence of ganglion cells in the submucosal plexus.

9   Which of the following statements regarding cystic fibrosis (CF) are *true*?

a CF is inherited in an autosomal dominant fashion.

b Ten per cent of infants with CF will suffer from meconium ileus leading to bowel obstruction.

c An abnormal sweat test is the gold standard for diagnosis, as it will always be positive in CF.

d Raised concentrations of immunoreactive trypsinogen in a Guthrie blood spot test helps identify infants who need further testing for CF.

e CF has been associated with congenital bilateral absence of the vas deferens in men.

10 Which of the following is a rare presentation of metabolic alkalosis in CF?

a Pyloric stenosis

b Milk-alkali syndrome

c Undiagnosed diabetes

d Imerslund–Gräsbeck syndrome

e Pseudo-Bartter's syndrome

Bibliography

American Academy of Pediatrics Committee on Environmental Health. Lead exposure in children: prevention, detection, and management. *Pediatrics*. 2005 Oct; **116**(4): 1036–46.

Bekkali NL, van den Berg MM, Dijkgraaf MG, *et al*. Rectal fecal impaction treatment in childhood constipation: enemas versus high doses oral PEG. *Pediatrics*. 2009 Dec; **124**(6): e1108–15.

Biggs WS, Dery WH. Evaluation and treatment of constipation in infants and children. *Am Fam Physician*. 2006 Feb 1; **73**(3): 469–77.

Binns HJ, Campbell C, Brown MJ; Centers for Disease Control and Prevention Advisory Committee on Childhood Lead Poisoning Prevention. Interpreting and managing blood lead levels of less than 10 microg/dL in children and reducing childhood exposure to lead: recommendations of the Centers for Disease Control and Prevention Advisory Committee on Childhood Lead Poisoning Prevention. *Pediatrics*. 2007 Nov; **120**(5): e1285–98.

British Medical Association; Royal Pharmaceutical Society of Great Britain.

British National Formulary. 61st ed. London: BMJ Group and Pharmaceutical Press; 2011.

Candy D, Belsey J. Macrogol (polyethylene glycol) laxatives in children with functional constipation and faecal impaction: a systematic review. *Arch Dis Child.* 2009 Feb; **94**(2): 156–60. Epub 2008 Nov 19.

Davies JC, Alton EW, Bush A. Cystic fibrosis. *BMJ.* 2007 Dec 15; **335**(7632): 1255–9.

El-Hodhod MA, Younis NT, Zaitoun YA, *et al.* Cow's milk allergy related pediatric constipation: appropriate time of milk tolerance. *Pediatr Allergy Immunol.* 2010 Mar; **21**(2 Pt. 2): e407–12. Epub 2009 Jun 25.

Iacono G, Carroccio A, Cavataio F, *et al.* Chronic constipation as a symptom of cow milk allergy. *J Pediatr.* 1995 Jan; **126**(1): 34–9.

Iacono G, Cavataio F, Montalto G, *et al.* Intolerance of cow's milk and chronic constipation in children. *N Engl J Med.* 1998 Oct 15; **339**(16): 1100–4.

Issenman RM, Filmer RB, Gorski PA. A review of bowel and bladder control development in children: how gastrointestinal and urologic conditions relate to problems in toilet training. *Pediatrics.* 1999 Jun; **103**(6 Pt. 2): 1346–52.

Kennedy JD, Dinwiddie R, Daman-Willems C, *et al.* Pseudo-Bartter's syndrome in cystic fibrosis. *Arch Dis Child.* 1990 Jul; **65**(7): 786–7.

Kiely EM, Chopra R, Corkery JJ. Delayed diagnosis of congenital anal stenosis. *Arch Dis Child.* 1979 Jan; **54**(1): 68–70.

Loening-Baucke V, Miele E, Staiano A. Fiber (glucomannan) is beneficial in the treatment of childhood constipation. *Pediatrics.* 2004 Mar; **113**(3 Pt. 1): e259–64.

MacKinlay GA, Watson ACH. Surgical pediatrics. In: Campbell AGM, McIntosh N, editors. *Forfar and Arneil's Textbook of Pediatrics.* 5th ed. New York, NY: Churchill Livingstone; 1998. pp. 1768–801.

Melendez E, Goldstein AM, Sagar P, *et al.* Case 3-2012: A newborn boy with vomiting, diarrhea, and abdominal distension. *N Engl J Med.* 2012; **366**: 361–72.

McKenzie S, Silverman M. Respiratory disorders. In: Campbell AGM, McIntosh N, editors. *Forfar and Arneil's Textbook of Pediatrics.* 5th ed. New York, NY: Churchill Livingstone; 1998. pp. 489–583.

National Collaborating Centre for Women's and Children's Health; National

Institute for Health and Clinical Excellence. *Constipation in Children and Young People; clinical guideline 99*. London: RCOG Press; 2010. http://guidance.nice.org.uk/CG99/Guidance/pdf/English

Olness K, Tobin J Sr. Chronic constipation in children: can it be managed by diet alone? *Postgrad Med*. 1982 Oct; **72**(4): 149–54.

Urinary tract infection

Eighteen-month-old Emma is seen in clinic by your colleague. Emma has a 12-hour history of fever, but she is well in herself and playful in clinic. A temperature of 38.6°C is noted. General examination is normal. Your colleague suspects the beginnings of a viral infection and advises accordingly. Later that evening Emma develops a temperature of 40°C and mum takes her to the local out-of-hours (OOH) GP. He also notes that Emma is well in herself. He advises mum to get a urine sample from Emma by packing her nappy with cotton wool balls and squeezing the urine into a clean container. After a few hours of persistence, mum manages to get a urine sample. Urine dipstick is positive for leucocyte esterase and negative for nitrite. Emma is commenced on an oral cephalasporin and she makes an uneventful recovery over the next 48 hours. Mum returns to see your colleague about the possibility of starting prophylactic antibiotics for Emma. He advises mum that this is not necessary. Unsatisfied, she sees you for a second opinion. A glance through Emma's notes suggests that she has been fairly well since her birth with no previous history of urinary tract infections (UTIs). There is no significant urological family history either.

Which of the following statements are *false*?

a A UTI should always be considered as a potential diagnosis in a febrile infant with no recognisable source of infection.

b The method of urine collection employed by the OOH GP is recommended because of its non-invasive nature and low rates of false positives.

c An ultrasound scan (USS) of the urinary tract should be performed in all children following their first UTI.

d A negative nitrite test on urine dipstick does not rule out a UTI, particularly if the child has frequently been emptying his or her bladder.

e A family history of vesicoureteric reflux (VUR) is an important determinant in the future management of the child.

f Asymptomatic bacteriuria should be aggressively treated, especially in female infants, because of the risk of pyelonephritis and renal scarring.

g Parental reporting of foul-smelling urine increases the risk of a UTI in a child.

Answer: b, c and f

UTIs are an important differential in the list of potential diagnoses in a febrile child. A UTI should always be considered in a febrile child with no obvious focus of infection. Acutely, UTIs can cause serious bacteraemia, particularly in infants. Prior to the availability of antibiotics, UTIs were potentially fatal. Now, there is greater interest in the potential long-term consequences of UTIs and how they can be avoided. The understanding of VUR and how it may be related to kidney damage and long-term complications has shaped the management of UTIs. VUR refers to the retrograde movement of urine from the bladder towards the kidneys. The damage done to the kidney by this abnormal flow, in the form of scarring, is termed reflux nephropathy. Whereas prospective studies have failed to consistently show a strong relation between reflux nephropathy and long-term complications, retrospective studies have linked renal scarring secondary to UTIs with later development of chronic kidney disease, hypertension and pre-eclampsia. Since retrospective trials look mainly at children who are being seen in tertiary centres (hence are likely to have suffered from recurrent infections and have significant reflux nephropathy), it would be unwise to extrapolate this data to apply to children with uncomplicated febrile UTIs who make uneventful recoveries in primary care.

The conclusion reached by the first doctor who saw Emma was not unreasonable. A well child presenting early with a fever may very well be at the initial stages of a viral infection. However, if the fever persists, without any obvious source of infection, the urine should be tested. Fever, abdominal pain (with or without loin pain), vomiting, reduced oral intake and generalised lethargy and irritability are common symptoms in infants with a UTI. Older children may complain of dysuria. Parental reporting of malodorous urine has been linked with an increased probability of a UTI (Gauthier, *et al.*, 2012; Couture, *et al.*, 2003). The urine collection method employed by the OOH doctor is not recommended. National Institute for Health and Care Excellence (NICE) guidelines suggest the use of a clean-catch urine sample. This can be quite a laborious process in which urine is collected directly into a clean container after cleaning the genital and perineal area to avoid contamination. Urine collection pads or bags may be used if a clean-catch sample is difficult to obtain. Although the use of pads or bags is much easier and more convenient, they are associated with higher contamination rates than clean-catch samples (Alam, *et al.*, 2005). Studies (Tosif, *et al.*, 2012; Hardy, *et al.*, 1976) have shown suprapubic aspiration and specimens from urinary catheterisation to be the least prone to bacterial contamination; however, they are much more invasive methods. If pads or bags are used, manufacturer instructions on their use should be followed. The perineum and genitalia should be cleaned prior to application and the pad or bag should be regularly changed, until a sample is collected, to avoid contamination. NICE guidelines specifically advise against the use of cotton wool balls, gauze and sanitary towels.

Ideally, the urine sample should be sent for urgent microscopy. Since this may not always be possible (particularly in an OOH setting), urinalysis with urine dipsticks is a useful way to ascertain the presence of a UTI. Since parents may be sent home with instructions on how to collect the sample, it is important they are made aware of how to store it also. If, after collection, the urine is kept at room temperature, urinalysis should be performed within an hour. This time period can be extended up to 4 hours on a refrigerated sample. The sample should be obtained prior to starting any treatment and should be sent for microscopy and culture after urinalysis. For the purposes of culture, the sample should be refrigerated or preserved with boric acid (one would need to follow guidelines of the local microbiology laboratory). Urine dipsticks are analysed for the presence of blood, leucocyte esterase and urinary nitrite. Leucocyte esterase is an indicator of pyuria (the presence of white blood cells in the urine) and is a highly sensitive (>90%) test, as the absence of pyuria in children with UTI is rare. However, since pyuria is common with other conditions (e.g. fever from other conditions, exercise), it has a lower specificity (around 70%). Urinary nitrite test is not a particularly sensitive test in children, as it requires the conversion of dietary nitrates into nitrites in the bladder by bacteria. Since this process takes about 4 hours, children who frequently empty their bladder will produce a negative nitrite test. Another reason for the nitrite test to be negative would be the presence of bacteria that do not reduce nitrate to nitrite. A positive test, though, helps confirm the diagnosis because of its high specificity. Asymptomatic bacteriuria is distinguished by the absence of pyuria. It does not need treating. Kemper and Avner (1992) concluded that screening for it is expensive and treating it does not reduce the risk of renal scarring and pyelonephritis. Asymptomatic bacteriuria should not be treated in children, as it is of uncertain benefit.

Treatment of an acute episode depends upon the clinical condition of the child. In this case it seems appropriate to have treated the child with oral antibiotics. If the child appears toxic and unwell, he or she should be referred to a paediatrician. NICE guidelines suggest that an infant younger than 3 months old with a febrile UTI should be treated with parenteral antibiotics. Interestingly, a recent study (Montini, *et al.*, 2007) compared oral co-amoxiclav with parenteral ceftriaxone in children with a first febrile UTI and found that they were equally effective. Their study included infants older than 1 month. However, extremely unwell children with suspected sepsis and those with known renal tract abnormalities were excluded from the study. Parenteral therapy should be considered in unwell children who are dehydrated or vomiting. If oral antibiotics are used, NICE suggests a 7- to 10-day course. Antimicrobial sensitivity data should be available from the local microbiology laboratory and an antibiotic with a low-resistance pattern should be used. Prophylactic antibiotics should not be started after a first febrile UTI but may be considered if infection is recurring. The degree of VUR, determined by imaging, may help decide which children would benefit from prophylactic antibiotics. VUR is classified as grade I–V, ranging from reflux into a non-dilated ureter to reflux into a grossly dilated renal tract with loss of papillary impressions in the kidney. Prophylactic antibodies may help children with VUR of grade III and above, as the risk of recurrent infection is greater in these children. Further studies are needed to help determine the optimal duration of prophylaxis. NICE guidelines do not routinely recommend surgical treatments for VUR. Surgical techniques include open reimplantation of the ureter (more effective) and endoscopic injections of bulking agents near the vesicoureteral junction. Surgery may be an option in children who continue to get febrile UTIs on different prophylactic antibiotics – hence, necessitating a specialist opinion from a paediatric urologist.

Rather than prophylactic antibiotics, the importance of prevention should be discussed with the mother. A careful history should rule out constipation. If concomitant constipation exists then this should be treated. An adequate fluid intake and appropriate genital hygiene should be encouraged. Inadequate and dysfunctional voiding has also been linked with recurrent UTIs. A history of this should be sought and appropriate advice given. Cranberry juice is widely recommended in women as prophylaxis against UTIs. It is thought to prevent the adhesion of microbes to the epithelial cells of the urinary tract. Studies in children are limited and inconclusive. Moreover, the amount of cranberry juice that would have to be ingested to prevent UTIs is unclear. If the child finds it palatable, it may be recommended. Circumcision in boys has been associated with a lower risk of UTI and may be considered in boys at a high risk of a UTI or with high-grade VUR (Singh-Grewal, et al., 2005).

Examination practice: urinary tract infection

Options for questions 11–13:

a   ultrasound during the acute infection (urgent)

b   ultrasound within 6 weeks of the infection (routine)

c   computed tomography scan of the renal tract within 6 weeks of infection

d   magnetic resonance imaging of the kidneys within 4 weeks of infection

e   micturating cystourethrogram

f   renal scintigraphy with dimercaptosuccinic acid (DMSA) at time of infection

g   renal scintigraphy with DMSA 4–6 months after the infection

h   options a and g

i   options b and g

j   none of the above.

Questions 11–13 describe children presenting with their mothers. Choose the correct form of imaging that the child should have as part of his or her management, according to NICE guidelines, from the list of options provided. Each answer may be chosen once, more than once or not at all.

11 A 4-month-old girl presents with fever and lethargy. Urine culture grows *Escherichia coli*. Oral antibiotics are started and she responds well to treatment within 48 hours and makes an uneventful recovery.

12 A 5-year-old boy presents to you with symptoms suggestive of a UTI. This is the third time this year. On previous occasions he made a quick recovery with oral antibiotics. He is well in himself but has a fever.

13 A 1-year-old girl presents with fever and severe dehydration. She is referred to the duty paediatric team for assessment. She is deemed to be septicaemic and is started on intravenous cephalosporins and fluids. Urine obtained from suprapubic aspiration grows *E. coli* upon culture. On day three she is switched to oral co-amoxiclav on advice from the microbiologist. She continues to have a low-grade fever but it settles on day five. She is discharged on day seven with a further week course of oral antibiotics.

14 Which of the following statements regarding antibiotic use in children is/are *correct*?

a   High-dose short-course amoxicillin treatment has been shown to reduce the spread of drug-resistant pneumococcus.

b   Up to 90% of patients presenting with a sore throat are likely to be symptom-free at 1 week, whether treated with antibiotics or not.

c   An uncomplicated lower UTI in a child should be treated for 10–14 days.

d   Chronic suppurative otitis media should always be treated with oral antibiotics, because of the higher antibiotic concentrations required in the middle ear to treat it.

e   Current guidance recommends antibiotic courses of greater than 3 weeks for osteomyelitis.

15 Which of the following is a non-neurotoxic option for the treatment of head lice?

a   Malathion

b   Dimeticone

c   Permethrin

d   Carbaryl

e   Ivermectin

Bibliography

Alam MT, Coulter JB, Pacheco J, *et al.* Comparison of urine contamination rates using three different methods of collection: clean-catch, cotton wool pad and urine bag. *Ann Trop Paediatr.* 2005 Mar; **25**(1): 29–34.

Campbell WC, Fisher MH, Stapley EO, *et al.* Ivermectin: a potent new antiparasitic agent. *Science.* 1983 Aug 26; **221**(4613): 823–8.

Cormican M, Murphy AW, Vellinga A. Interpreting asymptomatic bacteriuria. *BMJ.* 2011 Aug 4; **343**: d4780.

Couture E, Labbé V, Cyr C. Clinical predictors of positive urine cultures in young children at risk for urinary tract infection. *Paediatr Child Health.* 2003 Mar; **8**(3): 145–9.

de Bont EGPM, Francis NA, Dinant G, *et al.* Parents' knowledge, attitudes, and practice in childhood fever: an internet-based survey. *Br J Gen Pract.* 2014 Jan; **64**: 20–1.

Del Mar CB, Glasziou PP, Spinks AB. Antibiotics for sore throat. *Cochrane Database Syst Rev*. 2006 Oct 18; (4): CD000023.

Diamond DA, Mattoo TK. Endoscopic treatment of primary vesicoureteral reflux. *N Engl J Med*. 2012 Mar 29; **366**(13): 1218–26.

Gauthier M, Gouin S, Phan V, *et al*. Association of malodorous urine with urinary tract infection in children aged 1 to 36 months. *Pediatrics*. 2012 May; **129**(5): 885–90. Epub 2012 Apr 2.

Goldman RD. Cranberry juice for urinary tract infection in children. *Can Fam Physician*. 2012 Apr; **58**(4): 398–401.

Hardy JD, Furnell PM, Brumfitt W. Comparison of sterile bag, clean catch and suprapubic aspiration in the diagnosis of urinary infection in early childhood. *Br J Urol*. 1976 Aug; **48**(4): 279–83.

Kemper KJ, Avner ED. The case against screening urinalyses for asymptomatic bacteriuria in children. *Am J Dis Child*. 1992 Mar; **146**(3): 343–6.

Kerrison C, Riordan FA. How long should we treat this infection for? *Arch Dis Child Educ Pract Ed*. 2013 Aug; **98**(4): 136–40. Epub 2013 Jun 1.

Montini G, Toffolo A, Zucchetta P, *et al*. Antibiotic treatment for pyelonephritis in children: multicentre randomised controlled non-inferiority trial. *BMJ*. 2007 Aug 25; **335**(7616): 386. Epub 2007 Jul 4.

Montini G, Tullus K, Hewitt I. Febrile urinary tract infections in children. *N Engl J Med*. 2011 Jul 21; **365**(3): 239–50.

National Institute for Health and Care Excellence. *Urinary Tract Infection in Children: NICE clinical guideline 54*. London: NICE; 2007. www.nice.org.uk/CG54

Schlager TA. Urinary tract infections in children younger than 5 years of age: epidemiology, diagnosis, treatment, outcomes and prevention. *Paediatr Drugs*. 2001; **3**(3): 219–27.

Schrag SJ, Peña C, Fernández J, *et al*. Effect of short-course, high-dose amoxicillin therapy on resistant pneumococcal carriage: a randomized trial. *JAMA*. 2001 Jul 4; **286**(1): 49–56.

Singh-Grewal D, Macdessi J, Craig J. Circumcision for the prevention of urinary tract infection in boys: a systematic review of randomised trials and observational studies. *Arch Dis Child*. 2005 Aug; **90**(8): 853–8. Epub 2005 May 12.

Subcommittee on Urinary Tract Infection, Steering Committee on Quality

Improvement and Management, Roberts KB. Urinary tract infection: clinical practice guideline for the diagnosis and management of the initial UTI in febrile infants and children 2 to 24 months. *Pediatrics*. 2011 Sep; **128**(3): 595–610.

Tebruegge M, Pantazidou A, Curtis N. What's bugging you? An update on the treatment of head lice infestation. *Arch Dis Child Educ Pract Ed*. 2011 Feb; **96**(1): 2–8. Epub 2010 Aug 5.

Tosif S, Baker A, Oakley E, *et al.* Contamination rates of different urine collection methods for the diagnosis of urinary tract infections in young children: an observational cohort study. *J Paediatr Child Health*. 2012 Aug; **48**(8): 659–64. Epub 2012 Apr 27.

Atopic eczema

Mum and dad present with 2-year-old Josh. Last year he was diagnosed with atopic eczema after presenting to the practice with a typical-looking rash on his cheeks and extensor surfaces of his arms and legs. You note that he was prescribed some emollients and low-potency topical steroids. His parents consulted two separate doctors at later dates, when stronger steroids and alternative emollients were prescribed. They return with Josh in pretty much the same state as last year. They do not feel that the prescribed medication has made any difference to his condition. They are not sure if they are using the various creams and ointments appropriately. They have brought the various tubes and tubs they have been prescribed over the preceding months. You note that most are fairly full, with only small quantities used from each one.

Which of the following statements regarding atopic eczema are *true*?

a Soaps and detergents are common trigger factors for atopic eczema.

b Delaying solid food introduction till the age of 1 year has been shown to significantly reduce the risk of developing atopic eczema.

c If an older sibling suffers from atopic eczema, a strict exclusion diet should be encouraged in the lactating mother to prevent a recurrence in the breastfeeding infant.

d If topical antibiotics are used in an infective flare-up, their use should be limited to 2 weeks to prevent the development of resistance.

e Diluted bleach baths may be useful in managing children prone to skin infection.

Answer: a, d and e

Atopic eczema is a common childhood disorder, accounting for frequent visits to the doctor. Patient (if old enough) and parent education forms a cornerstone in the management of atopic eczema. Parents should be made aware that efforts are focused towards managing rather than curing the condition. Any misconceptions about the various treatment modalities should be dispelled at an early stage to ensure adequate control of the condition. Reassurance should be given that in the majority of cases the condition is self-limiting and resolves by the time the child reaches his or her mid-teens. The physical and psychological effects of the condition on the child and parents should be acknowledged and appropriate support should be offered.

Atopic eczema is diagnosed on the basis of the presence of a typical rash associated with itching. Younger children may have the typical rash on the extensor surfaces (rather than the usual flexural surfaces) and the cheeks. A history of atopy in the child or in a first-degree relative helps aid the diagnosis. The underlying mechanisms in atopic eczema have been probed extensively. The two major causative factors are considered to be a defective skin barrier function and skin inflammation. The breakdown in the skin defensive mechanisms, through a variety of mechanisms, is thought to increase the likelihood of allergen absorption and infection with microbial colonisation. Filaggrin gene defects have recently been identified as one of the underlying mechanisms increasing the risk of developing atopic eczema and asthma via altered skin barrier function (van den Oord and Sheikh, 2009). Cutaneous inflammation is triggered and maintained by a whole host of pro-inflammatory cytokines. Various inflammatory mediators are implicated and are serving as markers for research and future targeted drug development.

Atopic eczema may not always have a trigger. However if the history is strongly suggestive of a particular trigger then this should be avoided. Not uncommonly, parents will implicate various foods in the development of eczema. Cow's milk, eggs, nut, wheat, fish and soy have been implicated in atopic eczema in children. If the suspicion of food (or other) allergy is strong then allergy testing is justified. Alternatives to cow's milk and soy milk are sometimes necessary and formulas containing hydrolysed and elemental proteins are appropriate in such a scenario. Other milks (such as rice and almond) have insufficient protein and hence are not suitable for younger children and may occasionally cause severe harm (Keller, *et al.*, 2012). Parents may enquire about delaying introduction of solid foods into the diet to avoid the development of eczema, particularly in subsequent children. There is a possibility that an introduction of a varied diet within the first 4 months of life may be associated with an increased risk of developing eczema. There is no evidence that withholding solids beyond the age of 6 months is beneficial in preventing the condition (Zutavern, *et al.*, 2008). Mum should be advised that there is good evidence to recommend breastfeeding for the first 4 months of life, as this has been associated with a reduced risk of developing atopic eczema. Dietary restrictions during pregnancy and lactation have not been associated with a beneficial effect so should not be recommended.

Excellent skin care is crucial in maintaining prolonged flare-free periods. This is achieved with the regular application of emollients. Emollients are the mainstay in treating atopic eczema and parents should be made aware that their application is necessary even when the skin is clear. A large selection of emollients is available for prescription and range from greasy products (paraffin based) to creams and lotions that contain more water, allowing more cosmetically acceptable application. Their purpose is to retain moisture in the skin and directly hydrate the top surface also. Greasy, lipophilic ointments are more occlusive and, hence, trap more moisture than the more hydrophilic preparations. The former may, however, exacerbate acne and folliculitis, making them less acceptable in day-to-day use. It is important that the correct method and amount of application of emollients is explained to patients. Emollients should be applied frequently and in appropriate quantities. If the majority of the body is affected, a 500 g tub of emollient should not last for more than a month if applied appropriately. The emollient should be smoothed into the skin in the direction of hair growth and not rubbed in, as rubbing hinders absorption and increases the risk of folliculitis. If the child is washed prior to emollient application, the skin should be dabbed dry (rather than rubbed dry, as this is akin to scratching the skin) followed by emollient application. In school-going children, emollients should be available to use at school during the day to ensure adequate skin hydration. Parents should be advised that no one emollient is better than the other. The important thing is to find the best one for the child and to apply it frequently. The physician should be on the lookout for sensitivity to emollients, as some children may react to certain emollients. Aqueous cream, in particular, has been implicated in a high proportion of children developing skin reactions after application (Cork, *et al.*, 2003); therefore, aqueous cream should not be used as a leave-on emollient but is appropriate to use as a soap substitute. Many emollients are also available as bath additive preparations (such as oils and shower gels), which can be used to improve skin hydration and as alternatives to soaps.

Topical corticosteroids have been in use for many years and provide effective control against eczema flare-ups. It is not uncommon for parents to become worried upon the prescription of steroids resulting in non-compliance with treatment. When used properly, local and systemic side effects from steroids are uncommon. Parents should be informed that the effects of uncontrolled eczema (e.g. distress caused to the child, cutaneous infection) warrant the use of topical corticosteroids, despite the potential of adverse effects from their use. Depending on their potency, topical corticosteroids may be classified as mild, moderate, potent and very potent. Different clinicians may vary in their management of eczema. Some may use longer courses of milder steroids, whereas others are more inclined to give short bursts of greater-potency steroids. Parents should be made aware of a fingertip unit (FTU), which is a standard measure (the amount of steroid from the tip of an adult's finger to the first crease) for determining the amount of steroid cream or ointment that needs to be applied. Mum can be advised that the appropriate amount for Josh would be 2 FTUs for the leg and foot, 2 FTUs for the chest and abdomen, 3 FTUs for the back and buttocks and 1.5 FTUs each for the face and neck and the arm and hand. A reduced amount would be used in an infant, whereas more FTUs would be needed for an older, and hence larger, child. Since the face, neck and genitalia are slightly more sensitive than the rest of the body, it is more appropriate to use mild potency steroids here. Topical calcineurin inhibitors, pimecrolimus and tacrolimus are newer agents also directed against various mediators of the inflammatory response. They can be used in immunocompetent children (2 years of age and above) as 'steroid-sparing' agents. Their use is justified when there is a risk of developing side effects from excessive steroid use or from them being ineffectual. Although some data on long-term use are available (4 years for tacrolimus), caution should be exercised because of their relatively new nature and they should be prescribed for short-term treatment only. There are some concerns regarding the development of skin malignancies, necessitating advice to limit exposure to sunlight and sun lamps (Breuer, *et al.*, 2005).

Other measures in the management of atopic eczema include wet wraps, antihistamines, phototherapy and systemic immunosuppressant therapy. Wet wraps are a cumbersome but effective method in helping control the itching and dryness associated with atopic eczema. Steroid and/or emollient is applied on the skin with a wet bandage applied on top to help trap moisture in the skin and prevent itching by the child. The wet bandage is then covered with a dry bandage. The child should be kept in a warm environment because of the risk of getting cold overnight as the water evaporates. Sedating antihistamines may be used if itching is severely impairing sleep. It is also important to be on the lookout for infections. Bacterial, particularly staphylococcal, infections are often responsible for sudden flare-ups of eczema. Topical antibiotics may be used if the area of infection is localised. If large parts of the body are affected then systemic antibiotics should be considered. If recurrent skin infections are a problem then emollients containing antimicrobials may be used to reduce the risk of infection. Diluted bleach baths are similar to swimming in a chlorinated pool. A small amount of bleach is added to a full tub and the child is soaked in the water for approximately 10 minutes followed by rinsing of the skin with fresh water.

Examination practice: asthma

Options for questions 16–18:

a inhaled short-acting β₂-agonist as required

b addition of inhaled corticosteroids at a dose of 200 mcg/day

c addition of inhaled corticosteroids at a dose of 400 mcg/day

d addition of inhaled long-acting β₂-agonist as required

e inhaled ipratropium bromide via oxygen-driven nebuliser

f intravenous magnesium sulphate

g reduce dose of inhaled corticosteroids

h addition of inhaled nedocromil sodium

i none of the above.

Questions 16–18 refer to management of children with asthma presenting to your GP surgery. Choose the most suitable management option available from the options provided. Each answer may be used once, more than once or not at all.

16 A 3-year-old boy presents with shortness of breath. He has a respiratory rate of 30 and a pulse rate of 130. He is able to talk. Widespread wheeze is noted on auscultation. Short-acting β₂-agonist is given via a nebuliser, which results in temporary relief. However, he is struggling with his breathing again an hour later.

17 A 1-year-old boy is noted to wheeze, with minimal distress, over the winter months with an upper respiratory tract infection. He is currently not on any medication.

18 A 4-year-old girl is currently on 4 mg montelukast daily and uses a short-acting β₂-agonist when needed. Inhaled corticosteroids were stopped after two separate attempts because of a worsening cough and recurrent oral candidiasis. Her asthma remains poorly controlled.

19 Which of the following statements regarding eczema herpeticum are *false*?

   a Most cases of eczema herpeticum are caused by herpes zoster virus.

   b Recurrent episodes of eczema herpeticum are uncommon.

   c All children should be treated with intravenous antiviral treatment.

d   Antibiotic treatment is usually required to treat bacterial super-infection.

e   Untreated, eczema herpeticum is potentially fatal.

20 Which of the following formulas is correct when calculating mid-parental height (MPH) for estimation of final expected height in a boy?

a   MPH = {(Father's height + 14) + Mother's height} divided by 2

b   MPH = {(Father's height − 14) + Mother's height} divided by 2

c   MPH = {Father's height + (Mother's height + 14)} divided by 2

d   MPH = {Father's height + (Mother's height − 14)} divided by 2

e   None of the above

Bibliography

Breuer K, Werfel T, Kapp A. Safety and efficacy of topical calcineurin inhibitors in the treatment of childhood atopic dermatitis. *Am J Clin Dermatol*. 2005; **6**(2): 65–77.

British Thoracic Society; Scottish Intercollegiate Guidelines Network. *British Guideline on the Management of Asthma: a national clinical guideline*. Guideline no. 101. Edinburgh: Scottish Intercollegiate Guidelines Network; 2008 (revised January 2012). Available at www.sign.ac.uk/pdf/sign101.pdf (accessed 14 January 2014).

Cates CJ, Crilly JA, Rowe BH. Holding chambers (spacers) versus nebulisers for beta-agonist treatment of acute asthma. *Cochrane Database Syst Rev*. 2006 Apr 19; (2): CD000052.

Cork MJ, Timmins J, Holden C, *et al*. An audit of adverse drug reactions to aqueous cream in children with atopic eczema. *Pharm J*. 2003; **271**(7277): 747–8.

Dattani MT, Preece MA. Physical growth and development. In: Campbell AGM, McIntosh N, editors. *Forfar and Arneil's Textbook of Pediatrics*. 5th ed. New York, NY: Churchill Livingstone; 1998. pp. 349–80.

David TJ, Longson M. Herpes simplex infections in atopic eczema. *Arch Dis Child*. 1985 April; **60**(4): 338–43.

Heratizadeh A, Wichmann K, Werfel T. Food allergy and atopic dermatitis: how are they connected? *Curr Allergy Asthma Rep*. 2011 Aug; **11**(4): 284–91.

Keller MD, Shuker M, Heimall J, *et al*. Severe malnutrition resulting from use of rice milk in food elimination diets for atopic dermatitis. *Isr Med Assoc J.* 2012 Jan; **14**(1): 40–2.

Kneepkens CM, Brand PL. Clinical practice: breastfeeding and the prevention of allergy. *Eur J Pediatr.* 2010 Aug; **169**(8): 911–17.

Knorr B, Franchi LM, Bisgaard H, *et al.* Montelukast, a leukotriene receptor antagonist, for the treatment of persistent asthma in children aged 2 to 5 years. *Pediatrics.* 2001 Sep; **108**(3): E48.

Krakowski AC, Eichenfield LF, Dohil MA. Management of atopic dermatitis in the pediatric population. *Pediatrics.* 2008 Oct; **122**(4): 812–24.

Lewis-Jones S, Mugglestone MA. Management of atopic eczema in children aged up to 12 years: summary of NICE guidance. *BMJ.* 2007; **335**(7632): 1263–4.

Liddle BJ. Herpes simplex infections in atopic eczema. *Arch Dis Child.* 1990 March; **65**(3): 333.

Lin C-Y. *Eczema Herpeticum.* DermNet NZ; 2010. Available at: www.dermnetnz.org/viral/eczema-herpeticum.html (accessed 22 September 2013).

National Institute for Health and Care Excellence. *Atopic Eczema in Children: NICE clinical guideline 57.* London: NICE; 2007. http://guidance.nice.org.uk/CG57

Van den Oord RA, Sheikh A. Filaggrin gene defects and risk of developing allergic sensitisation and allergic disorders: systematic review and meta-analysis. *BMJ.* 2009 Jul 9; **339**: b2433.

Zutavern A, Brockow I, Schaaf B, *et al.* Timing of solid food introduction in relation to eczema, asthma, allergic rhinitis, and food and inhalant sensitization at the age of 6 years: results from the prospective birth cohort study LISA. *Pediatrics.* 2008 Jan; **121**(1): e44–52.

Acne

Fifteen-year-old Josh comes to see you in your clinic. He is the captain of the school basketball team. You note that he came to see your colleague 3 weeks ago complaining about his skin. Acne was diagnosed and a topical antibiotic was prescribed. He is clutching a piece of paper as he walks in today. He tells you that the antibiotic gel that he was prescribed did nothing for his skin. A friend of his saw a private dermatologist who had prescribed him a drug that had immediately cured his acne. He has the name of the drug scribbled on this piece of paper: isotretinoin. Josh requests that he be prescribed this for his acne also, as he is suffering from a lack of self-confidence due to the state of his skin. Close examination of the skin reveals four or five comedones scattered around the forehead. No other lesions are seen elsewhere and Josh's back and chest are also clear. The only other noticeable thing in his notes is that he was under the care of the paediatric mental health team 2 years ago because of self-harming behaviour after the death of his father from a myocardial infarction at the age of 50.

Which of the following statements is *true*?

a   Josh should be advised that his acne is not severe enough to warrant any treatment and that he should wait for it to settle on its own.

b Isotretinoin is contraindicated in Josh because of his past history of mental health problems.

c Isotretinoin may lead to permanent remission of the acne.

d Isotretinoin therapy may lower triglyceride levels.

e Women who fall pregnant on isotretinoin should be reassured that data from animal studies suggest that it is safe to take the drug up to the end of the first trimester.

Answer: c

Acne is among the commonest skin conditions affecting teenagers. It is a cause of considerable anxiety and psychological morbidity among sufferers. It is not uncommon in clinical practice to find some teenagers to be completely unbothered by severe widespread acne and others to be extremely distressed by a few spots scattered here and there. It is therefore important to consider the impact the condition has on the patient while formulating a management plan. By a series of questionnaires, Mallon, *et al.* (1999) demonstrated that the sufferers of severe acne may suffer from similar levels of psychological morbidity as diabetes, asthma and epilepsy sufferers. It is therefore important that Josh's plight is not trivialised despite the fact he may be suffering from mild acne.

Acne is characterised by the presence of comedones, which are non-inflammatory follicular lesions. The follicle may be open (blackheads) or closed (whiteheads). They may be the only lesions present or may be accompanied by inflamed papules, cysts and pustules. The more severe the acne, the larger, deeper and more inflamed are the lesions. In severe cases deep nodular lesions may develop that are filled with mucopurulent material and are more likely to scar. In a rare form of acne, acne conglobata, these nodules may interconnect and require drainage, resulting in an exceptionally severe form of disease.

Treatment of acne is determined by the severity of disease and may be topical or by oral medication. Some people may mistake blackheads for dirt and be excessive in their attempts to clean these lesions. They should be advised that blackheads are just open follicles, full of sebum and dead cells. Their black colour is due to the oxidisation of the melanin pigment. Excessive cleaning may result in skin irritation, making them less likely to tolerate some of the topical treatments discussed shortly. Once-a-day gentle scrubbing to remove dead cells and avoidance of application of oily substances (such as make-up) to the skin should help with simple comedonal lesions. However, clinicians who deal with acne on a daily basis will know that rarely will most teenagers be satisfied just with advice, as most will seek some form of treatment to help with the lesions.

In mild to moderate acne it is appropriate to start with topical treatment. Topical treatment may consist of antibacterials, retinoids, keratolytics or combination therapy. Antibacterials are targeted against *Propionibacterium acnes*, the chief coloniser of the pilosebaceous unit. Topical preparations of erythromycin and clindamycin may be used to treat inflammatory lesions. As with all topical treatments, skin irritation may occur. The primary problem with topical antibacterials is the development of antibacterial resistance. This is likely to demonstrate itself as a reduced clinical response to the topical preparations. To prevent resistance from developing, concomitant use with oral antibiotics and unnecessarily long uninterrupted courses should be avoided. Another way of avoiding the development of resistance is the simultaneous use of the anti-keratolytic benzoyl peroxide. Benzoyl peroxide is a powerful oxidising agent with antibacterial activity as well. When used with erythromycin, it has been shown to reduce the development of antibacterial resistance (Harkaway, *et al.*, 1992). Hence, combination treatment of the two or courses of topical antibacterial therapy broken with benzoyl peroxide use may be an effective way of treating acne while reducing the risk of the development of resistant bacterial strains. Azelaic acid is another anti-keratolytic agent with antibacterial activity, and one with the advantage of being less likely than benzoyl peroxide to cause skin irritation. Topical retinoids, which are vitamin A derivatives, have anti-comedonal and anti-inflammatory properties. Contact with mucous membranes and peeling skin should be avoided, as should exposure to ultraviolet light post application. Hence, they are usually applied at night. They are contraindicated in pregnant women because of the risk of embryopathy. Adapalene 0.1%, a topical retinoid, has been shown to be effective when used in combination with benzoyl peroxide 2.5% when compared with using either one of them alone. This combination has been shown to have an early onset of action and be effective against treating inflammatory and non-inflammatory lesions (Keating, 2011). Topical treatments should be prescribed for at least 3–6 months in order to see the full impact of their effect.

Oral options for Josh include antibiotics and retinoids. In females, hormonal treatment is another option. Oral antibiotics, with evidence of benefit include, erythromycin and the tetracyclines; tetracycline, oxytetracycline, doxycycline, minocycline and lymecycline. Resistance to erythromycin is becoming more common. If there is a lack of response or a flare-up while taking treatment, an alternative antibiotic should be sought. Tetracycline or oxytetracycline will generally be used as first line. They are used in twice-daily regimens and it is appropriate to wait for 3 months for a response. If adequate response is seen, treatment should continue for at least 6 months. In some cases it may be necessary to continue for 2 years. They are taken on an empty stomach, with particular avoidance of milk, which reduces their absorption. A lack of adequate response warrants a switch to one of the other tetracyclines. Doxycycline and lymecycline have the advantage of once-daily dosing; 100 and 408 mg daily, respectively. Minocycline is given at a dose of 100 mg once a day or 50 mg twice daily. All tetracyclines carry the risk of causing drug-induced lupus erythematosus, but the risk with minocycline is the highest. Tetracyclines are deposited in growing bone and teeth and hence should not be given to children under the age of 12 or during pregnancy and lactation. If there is a lack of response to two different antibiotics, and a switch to oral retinoids is being considered, trimethoprim may be considered as a third-line antibiotic. Its use in the context of acne is unlicensed but, at a dose of 300 mg twice daily, it has been shown to be effective and reasonably safe (Cunliffe, *et al.*, 1999). Prolonged use of trimethoprim has been associated with marrow suppression (not as likely as when used in combination with sulfamethoxazole). Isotretinoin, the oral retinoid licensed for use in acne, is the drug that Josh seems to be interested in because of the effects it had on his friend. Isotretinoin is more effective than the aforementioned treatment options but it also has the potential of more serious side effects. Isotretinoin not only stunts the growth of *P. acnes* but also reduces the size of the pilosebaceous unit and encourages normal follicular keratinisation. It is therefore effective against comedonal and inflammatory disease. The list of potential side effects is large but dryness of eyes, mucosa and skin should be warned against. Infections of the skin and mucosa should be monitored for. It has also been associated with raised triglyceride levels, raised serum cholesterol with a drop in high-density lipoprotein levels. This may be significant in Josh's case because of the young age at which his father suffered from a myocardial infarction. Cholesterol and trigylceride levels are routinely measured before and during isotretinoin therapy. Another important consideration is the association between isotretinoin use and depression, necessitating a mental health review during follow-up appointments (Azoulay, *et al.*, 2008). Although a concern, Josh's history of depression is not an absolute contraindication to the use of isotretinoin. Although isotretinoin therapy is initiated by dermatologists, it is important to be aware of the potential complications of treatment so that they may be readily recognised in primary care. Since the perceived severity by the patient is also important in how acne is managed, isotretinoin should be considered in patients if they are extremely distressed by it. Josh should be made aware of the potential side effects of the drug and the existence of alternatives that he has not yet tried and which are likely to produce the desired effect because of the mild nature of his condition. Regular reviews may be necessary to reassure him and to monitor effects of therapy.

Examination practice: childhood rashes

Options for questions 21–23:

a impetigo

b molluscum contagiosum

c pityriasis rosea

d erythema toxicum neonatorum

e papular acrodermatitis of childhood

f pediculosis capitis

g acrodermatitis enteropathica

h erythema marginatum

i pityriasis versicolor.

Questions 21–23 refer to children presenting with a rash. Choose the most likely diagnosis from the options provided. Each option may be used once, more than once or not at all.

21 A 12-year-old boy is seen with a widespread rash consisting of oval macules spread in a 'fir tree pattern' over the trunk. He is systemically well and reports a single lesion appearing on his neck 3 days prior to the widespread rash.

22 A 6-month-old girl with cystic fibrosis presents with an erythematous, crusted rash around the mouth and nose. Blood tests reveal negligible zinc levels.

23 A 3-year-old girl presents with a crop of pearly white, dome-shaped lesions just under her right armpit. Mum thinks they may have appeared since she started swimming at the local swimming pool.

24 Which of the following statements regarding haemangiomas is/are *true*?

a Haemangiomas are benign proliferative tumours of endothelial cells.

b They are usually present at birth, after which they go through a slow growth phase.

c They should always be treated upon identification because of the risk of haemorrhagic bleed.

d Oral or intralesional steroids may be used to help slow their growth.

e Sturge–Weber's syndrome describes a haemangioma of the face associated with a lesion on the ipsilateral meninges and cerebral cortex.

25 Congenital absence of the canal of Schlemm may result in which condition of the eye?

a Buphthalmos

b Infantile macular degeneration

c Congenital obstruction of the nasolacrimal duct

d Meibomian cyst

e Entropion

Bibliography

Azoulay L, Blais L, Koren G, *et al.* Isotretinoin and the risk of depression in patients with acne vulgaris: a case-crossover study. *J Clin Psychiatry.* 2008 Apr; **69**(4): 526–32.

Cant JS. Disorders of the eye. In: Campbell AGM, McIntosh N, editors. *Forfar and Arneil's Textbook of Pediatrics.* 5th ed. New York, NY: Churchill Livingstone; 1998. pp. 1649–78.

Cunliffe WJ, Aldana OL, Goulden V. Oral trimethoprim: a relatively safe and successful third-line treatment for acne vulgaris. *Br J Dermatol.* 1999 Oct; **141**(4): 757–8.

Goulden V. Guidelines for the management of acne vulgaris in adolescents. *Paediatr Drugs.* 2003; **5**(5): 301–13.

Harkaway KS, McGinley KJ, Foglia AN, *et al.* Antibiotic resistance patterns in coagulase-negative staphylococci after treatment with topical erythromycin, benzoyl peroxide, and combination therapy. *Br Dermatol.* 1992 Jun; **126**(6): 586–90.

Healy E, Simpson N. Acne vulgaris. *BMJ.* 1994; **308**(6932): 831–3.

James WD. Clinical practice: acne. *N Engl J Med.* 2005 Apr 7; **352**(14): 1463–72.

Keating GM. Adapalene 0.1%/benzoyl peroxide 2.5% gel: a review of its use in the treatment of acne vulgaris in patients aged ≥ 12 years. *Am J Clin Dermatol.* 2011 Dec 1; **12**(6): 407–20.

Mallon E, Newton JN, Klassen A, *et al.* The quality of life in acne: a comparison with general medical conditions using generic questionnaires. *Br J Dermatol.* 1999 Apr; **140**(4): 672–6.

Rogers M, Barnetson RSC. Diseases of the skin. In: Campbell AGM, McIntosh N, editors. *Forfar and Arneil's Textbook of Pediatrics*. 5th ed. New York, NY: Churchill Livingstone; 1998. pp. 1616–48.

Starkey E, Shahidullah H. Propranolol for infantile haemangiomas: a review. *Arch Dis Child*. 2011 Sep; **96**(9): 890–3. Epub 2011 May 28.

Stulberg DL, Wolfrey J. Pityriasis rosea. *Am Fam Physician*. 2004 Jan 1; **69**(1): 87–91.

Kawasaki disease

The last appointment in your morning emergency clinic is 3-year-old Emaan. Before you call her in, you decide to have a quick look at her notes and notice the following entries in chronological order over the last few days.

Day 1   Twelve-hour history of fever. Difficult to control with antipyretics. Reduced oral intake. O/e [on examination] appears well. Temperature 38.5°C. No rashes. No meningism. ENT [ear, nose and throat] and chest examination normal. Abdomen soft and non-tender. ? Start of viral infection. Advised to observe, push fluids and review if any concerns.

Day 2   High fever continues. Now developed conjunctivitis and achy joints. O/e well hydrated. Inflamed conjunctiva. Pharynx inflamed. Temperature 39.0°C. No meningism. Tender anterior cervical lymph nodes. No joint swelling. ? Bacterial infection. Script for phenoxymethylpenicillin 125 mg/5 mL. 5 mL four times a day.

Day 3   Developed rash within few hours of starting penicillin so mum stopped medicine. O/e morbilliform rash on abdomen and chest. Mild scarlatiniform rash on arms and legs. Throat remains injected and conjunctiva slightly improved. ? Scarlet fever. ? Reaction to penicillin. Throat swab taken and treatment switched to erythromycin. To be continued for 10 days.

Today is day five of the illness. You have the throat swab results in front of you, which read: *Throat swab; normal upper respiratory tract flora.*

As you call Emaan in you notice that the rash is still apparent on her body. Mum says the fever has persisted and she does not feel she is any better at all. You notice Emaan has cracked lips, a swollen red tongue, high fever and mild oedema of her hands and feet.

Which of the following statements regarding Kawasaki disease is/are *true*?
a   Kawasaki disease is a self-limiting condition.
b   Kawasaki disease is most common in the first 6 months of life, with a second peak in incidence after the sixth decade of life.
c   Management of Emaan was inappropriate, as she fulfilled the criteria for the diagnosis of Kawasaki disease on day three.
d   Effective treatment to prevent the coronary complications of Kawasaki disease is available.
e   Aspirin, during the febrile phase of the illness, is contraindicated in this child because of the risk of developing Reye's syndrome.

Answer: a and d

This case demonstrates how difficult it may be to make a correct diagnosis of a rare condition, particularly when it so often mimics much more commonly encountered conditions. Physicians should have a high index of suspicion and be extra vigilant of any rare condition that has the following triad of features: (1) mimics much commoner, less serious conditions, making diagnosis difficult; (2) has devastating complications; and (3) has effective treatment when diagnosed early (*see* Figure 1). Bacterial meningitis fits the bill for this triad and is usually what most parents and healthcare workers are concerned about. However, Kawasaki disease is an important diagnosis that needs to be considered in any child with a persistent fever, as it arguably fulfils the aforementioned trio of features more aptly. Kawasaki disease is a self-limiting vasculitis that can occur in children of any age. It is more common in children between the ages of 6 months and 5 years. In the absence of treatment, symptoms and signs will normally resolve over the course of

10 days. The exact cause of Kawasaki disease remains elusive. Infectious agents are frequently suggested as the cause, based on the seasonal peaks of Kawasaki disease in various geographical regions. This is supported by the fact that it is uncommon in children under the age of 3 months, suggesting a protective role of transplacental antibodies against the infectious agent. Bacterial toxins, behaving as superantigens, triggering an inflammatory cascade have also been suggested but have never been convincingly isolated in patients with the condition. Incidence in the UK is estimated at eight cases per 100 000 children under the age of 5. Increased recognition of the condition is thought to be responsible for the rising incidence (Harnden, *et al.*, 2002). Incidence is higher among Asians from the Indian subcontinent (Gardner-Medwin, *et al.*, 2002).

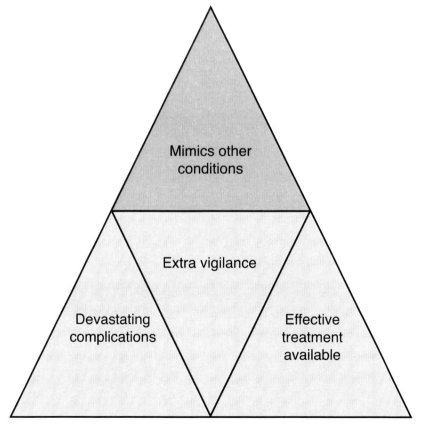

FIGURE 1

- **Mimics other conditions**: a diagnostic test for Kawasaki disease does not exist. Diagnosis is based on the presence of a persistent fever along with the presence of various clinical features. The fever has to be present for at least 5 days (hence option c is false) and four of the following five criteria should be present.

  1 *Bilateral conjunctival inflammation.* This is usually non-purulent and appears early in the illness and may therefore be mistaken for a viral conjunctivitis.

  2 *Oropharyngeal changes.* This may include cracked, fissured and inflamed lips, an inflamed, non-purulent pharynx and strawberry tongue. These, in combination with fever, can easily be mistaken for a viral infection. A strawberry tongue is commonly associated with scarlet fever.

  3 *A polymorphous rash.* The most non-specific of signs, the rash may be maculopapaular (morbilliform), consist of discrete lesions (erythema multiforme) or be scarlatiniform (diffusely distributed numerous red papules), hence compounding the chances of a misdiagnosis.

  4 *Cervical lymphadenopathy*, which may present in the form of a solitary lymph node. This can easily be confused for bacterial infection.

  5 *Changes in the extremities.* This may include oedema and erythema. Late in the illness, desquamation of the fingers and toes tends to take place.

These features tend not to appear together, making prompt diagnosis difficult. A high index of suspicion is required to make an accurate diagnosis, as the signs and symptoms unfold over the course of 5–10 days. Diagnostic accuracy is further made difficult by the presence of 'incomplete Kawasaki disease', in which only two of the five listed features may be present with persistent fever. Although not diagnostic, acute-phase reactants such as erythrocyte sedimentation rate and C-reactive protein will be raised. White blood cell count is also likely to be raised. These are worth measuring in the acute illness, as subsequent measurements may help monitor disease activity.

- **Devastating complications**: prompt diagnosis of Kawasaki disease is important, as a missed, untreated episode carries a significant risk of serious consequences for the child. The major cause of morbidity and, rarely, mortality, is due to cardiovascular complications, specifically related to coronary artery disease that occurs as a result of the vasculitic process. Although coronary artery changes are seen in up to half of children with the illness, these will regress in the majority of cases. Some, however, will proceed to form aneurysms that may stenose, thrombose or rupture. Worryingly, the dilatation of the coronary arteries may start within the first 2 weeks of developing fever. All children with a diagnosis of Kawasaki disease should have access to echocardiography in the acute phase of the illness, as it is a reliable method of detecting coronary artery aneurysms. It should be performed as soon as the diagnosis is suspected. Subsequent timings may be determined by the nature of the initial result. In uncomplicated cases further echocardiograms should be performed at 2 weeks and then 6–8 weeks from diagnosis. More frequent scans will be needed where complications are likely to develop (Newberger, et al., 2004). Other complications include myocarditis, pancarditis and, rarely, heart failure. Long-term complications of the condition remain to be elucidated. A cohort of over 3000 patients with Kawasaki disease in childhood is being followed up in Japan. Some patients in the cohort are reaching their fourth decade. The hope is that they will help unravel the true impact of this intriguing condition on those who survive it into adulthood.

- **Effective treatment**: a single infusion of intravenous immunoglobulin (IVIG), given at a dose of 2 g/kg, forms the mainstay of treatment of Kawasaki disease. It should be given between days five and ten of the illness, with the onset of fever marking day one of the illness. It is effective in reducing fever within 36 hours of administration and reduces the risk of developing coronary artery aneurysms significantly. It can and should be administered after day ten of the illness if the diagnosis was initially missed or if there is evidence of ongoing inflammation and fever. It is believed to work by having a generalised anti-inflammatory effect. Aspirin is used in conjunction with IVIG as an anti-inflammatory and antiplatelet agent. High doses are usually prescribed during the febrile phase, with a lower maintenance dose until a normal echocardiogram is seen at around 6 weeks. Aspirin does not appear to have a protective effect against the development of coronary artery disease. Other anti-inflammatory agents and treatment modalities that have been used in cases where fever persists despite IVIG include corticosteroids, plasmapharesis, cyclophosphamide, ciclosporin, ulinastatin (human trypsin inhibitor), abciximab (platelet glycoprotein IIb/IIIa receptor inhibitor) and infliximab (monoclonal antibodies against tumour necrosis factor-α).

Examination practice: eponymous syndromes

Options for questions 26–28:

a McArdle's syndrome

b Wilson's disease

c Von Gierke's disease

d Wolman's disease

e glucose-6-phosphate dehydrogenase deficiency

f Krabbe's disease

g Menkes's syndrome

h Dubin–Johnson syndrome

i Fanconi's syndrome.

Choose the most appropriate answer from the options provided for questions 26–28. Each option may be used once, more than once or not at all.

26 Low copper levels associated with kinky, steel-like hair, osteoporosis, developmental retardation and seizures.

27 Enzyme deficiency leads to failure to dephosphorylate glucose-6-phosphate, resulting in lack of glucose production and possible hypoglycaemia.

28 Muscle phosphorylase deficiency leads to easy fatigability during exercise.

29 Which of the following statements regarding congenital heart disease are *true*?

    a Ebstein's anomaly has been linked with maternal lithium ingestion during pregnancy.

    b A ventricular septal defect (VSD) is the commonest of the cyanotic congenital heart lesions.

    c Coarctation of the aorta occurs more frequently in girls with Turner's syndrome.

    d Dextrocardia refers to an anatomically abnormal heart, more than half of which lies in the right side of the chest.

    e Infants with tetralogy of Fallot are picked up at birth because of immediate cyanosis secondary to pulmonary stenosis.

30 Ten-year-old Joshua presents with mum who tells you that he has been complaining of left-sided chest pain for 2 weeks. On examination you find an isolated, tender and mildly swollen second costochondral junction. What is the most likely diagnosis?

a Costochondritis

b Tietze's syndrome

c Slipping rib syndrome

d Texidor's twinge

e Pericarditis

Bibliography

Buist NRM. Inborn errors of metabolism. In: Campbell AGM, McIntosh N, editors. *Forfar and Arneil's Textbook of Pediatrics.* 5th ed. New York, NY: Churchill Livingstone; 1998. pp. 1099–178.

Burns JC, Glodé MP. Kawasaki syndrome. *Lancet.* 2004 Aug 7–13; **364**(9433): 533–44.

Frank JE. Diagnosis and management of G6PD deficiency. *Am Fam Physician.* 2005 Oct 1; **72**(7): 1277–82.

Gardner-Medwin JM, Dolezalova P, Cummins C, *et al.* Incidence of Henoch-Schönlein purpura, Kawasaki disease, and rare vasculitides in children of different ethnic origins. *Lancet.* 2002 Oct 19; **360**(9341): 1197–202.

Gordon JB, Kahn AM, Burns JC. When children with Kawasaki disease grow up: myocardial and vascular complications in adulthood. *J Am Coll Cardiol.* 2009 Nov 17; **54**(21): 1911–20.

Harnden A, Alves B, Sheikh A. Rising incidence of Kawasaki disease in England: analysis of hospital admission data. *BMJ.* 2002 Jun 15; **324**(7351): 1424–5.

Harnden A, Takahashi M, Burgner D. Kawasaki disease. *BMJ.* 2009 May 5; **338**: b1514.

Houston AB. Cardiovascular disease. In: Campbell AGM, McIntosh N, editors. *Forfar and Arneil's Textbook of Pediatrics.* 5th ed. New York, NY: Churchill Livingstone; 1998. pp. 584–640.

Ives A, Daubeney PE, Balfour-Lynn IM. Recurrent chest pain in the well child. *Arch Dis Child.* 2010 Aug; **95**(8): 649–54. Epub 2010 Apr 6.

Newburger JW, Takahashi M, Gerber MA, *et al.* Diagnosis, treatment, and long-term management of Kawasaki disease: a statement for health professionals from the Committee on Rheumatic Fever, Endocarditis, and Kawasaki Disease, Council on Cardiovascular Disease in the Young, American Heart Association. *Pediatrics*. 2004 Dec; **114**(6): 1708–33.

Tidy C. *McArdle's Glycogen Storage Disease*. Leeds: Patient.co.uk, Egton Medical Information Systems Limited; 2011. Available at: www.patient.co.uk/doctor/mcardles-glycogen-storage-disease (accessed 5 June 2013).

Henoch–Schönlein purpura

The flu season is in full swing and you have already seen half a dozen kids whom you have diagnosed as having viral upper respiratory tract infections. Next on the list is 8-year-old Mark. He came to see you 3 days ago with mum, complaining of a runny nose, sore throat and mild cough. Examination had been unremarkable and a viral infection diagnosed. As he settles in the chair, you note that he appears generally well. Mum tells you that he has been complaining of intermittent abdominal pain since yesterday. He vomited twice yesterday but has had no episodes of vomiting today. More worryingly he has been complaining of pain in his knee joints, which has caused difficulty walking. You examine Mark's abdomen on the couch and note that, although soft on palpation, it is generally tender. As you are examining his knees, a purplish rash over the lateral aspect of his thighs catches your eyes. On closer inspection this extends over his buttocks and is raised and palpable. You suspect a diagnosis of Henoch–Schönlein purpura (HSP).

Which of the following statements is/are *false*?

a   A diagnosis of HSP cannot be made without a lumbar puncture, as bacterial meningitis needs to be excluded as a cause for the purpuric rash.

b   Abdominal pain and arthritis are cardinal features of HSP, occurring in practically all children with the condition.

c   Nine out of ten cases of HSP will occur in children under the age of 10.
d   IgG is strongly linked with the pathogenesis of the condition, with raised levels almost invariably seen.
e   The multisystem manifestations of HSP rarely settle spontaneously, necessitating steroid treatment in the majority of children.

Answer: all apart from c are false

HSP derives its name from the descriptions of the condition by Johann Schönlein and his student Eduard Henoch in the 1800s. HSP is a systemic vasculitis of unknown aetiology and is the commonest vasculitic condition of childhood. One study found the estimated annual incidence to be as high as 70.3/100 000 among children between the ages of 4 and 7 in the West Midlands (Gardner-Medwin, *et al.*, 2002). It is more common in boys. Many infectious pathogens (most commonly group A β-haemolytic streptococcus), immunisations and drugs have been suggested as infectious triggers of the condition but none have been firmly established as the cause. More recently it has been linked with influenza vaccinations during the pandemic of influenza A (H1N1) in 2009 (Watanabe, 2010). The large majority of cases are in children under the age of 10 but it may occur in adults also, where it may present atypically and in a more severe form. IgA (rather than IgG) is strongly linked with the immunopathogenesis of the condition, with IgA1 deposits found in the skin, gut and renal mesangium.

In the absence of a specific diagnostic test, diagnosis is based on presenting clinical features. Routine bloods (full blood count, urea, electrolytes and creatinine, clotting screen, liver function tests) and urinalysis should be performed as part of the initial work-up on presentation. Other tests such as an autoimmune profile and complement levels should be performed if the diagnosis is in doubt. Since the child with HSP is generally systemically well, a lumbar puncture to exclude bacterial meningitis is not necessary. However, if the diagnosis is unclear or the child is unwell, then other appropriate investigations to determine the source of infection will become necessary. Figure 2 lists the important clinical features of HSP.

As the name of the condition suggests, a purpuric rash is the cardinal

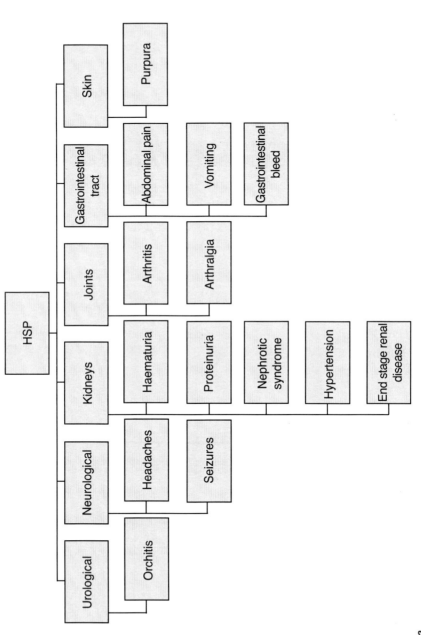

FIGURE 2

symptom that allows the diagnosis to be made, as it is present in all cases of HSP. However, it may appear after the onset of other signs and symptoms listed here, making diagnosis of HSP difficult (Mrusek, *et al.*, 2004). The rash may initially present as urticaria or erythematous maculopapular lesions progressing to a palpable purpura. Oedema and haemorrhage of the bowel, as a result of the vasculitic process, is responsible for the gastrointestinal symptoms. Occasionally HSP may cause severe abdominal pain, mimicking serious gastrointestinal pathology. Intussusception, perforation and obstruction are rare complications of HSP necessitating further investigations when suspected. The arthritis and arthralgia of HSP is particularly debilitating but does not result in lasting joint damage. Kidney involvement is the most important in terms of long-term sequelae of the condition. Renal manifestations of HSP almost always occur after the onset of the typical purpuric rash. Nephritis will occur in approximately 40% of HSP sufferers (Saulsbury, 2007) and will be manifest within 3 months in practically all cases. Hence, GPs should monitor blood pressure and urine (in the form of early morning urine dipstick) weekly in the first month of the illness. Thereafter, monitoring can be done fortnightly. If macroscopic haematuria, hypertension or proteinuria is detected, the child should be referred to a paediatrician. These children are likely to need long-term follow-up because of the potential for late deterioration of renal disease (Jauhola, *et al.*, 2012). In the absence of the above, less frequent monitoring should be continued. If after a year of the onset of illness blood pressure and urinalysis remain normal, the child and parents can be reassured that the risk of developing renal complications of the illness are very little and the child can be safely discharged from follow-up. If microscopic haematuria persists, yearly urine and blood pressure reviews should continue. Local guidelines may vary on the frequency of reviews needed and should always be referred to.

Treatment of HSP may be considered under two separate categories:

1   rapid relief of symptoms
2   prevention of long-term complications.

HSP is a self-limiting condition, recurring in approximately 33% of patients. In the majority of children, the disease will have subsided by 4 weeks. Bed rest with adequate hydration is generally recommended, as it helps with the resolution of the rash and oedema. Arthritic pain responds well to non-steroidal anti-inflammatory drugs; however, their use may be limited in the presence of renal disease. Abdominal pain can be distressing and may require opiate analgesia. If this fails, steroids are frequently employed to help with the pain. There is some evidence to support their use and they may also help with joint pain. There is no convincing evidence that steroids help with the skin manifestations of the disease, which rarely requires treatment anyway. The more important question is whether steroids should be used to help treat kidney involvement in HSP. Children who develop renal complications (nephritic or nephrotic syndrome and/or reduced renal function) are likely to have a poorer prognosis and recurrence of disease. Hence, debate and controversy continues on the role of treatment with steroids and other agents early on in the disease to prevent long-term renal complications. Corticosteroids, unfortunately, have not been shown to prevent the development of HSP-associated delayed nephritis. Despite the lack of evidence, those with severe renal disease are likely to be treated more aggressively because of the potential for adverse long-term consequences. Other agents used may include immunosuppresants such as cyclophosphamide, azathioprine or ciclosporin. This will normally involve the input of a paediatric nephrologist.

Examination practice: vitamin and mineral deficiencies

Options for questions 31–33:

a   vitamin A

b   vitamin D

c   vitamin B_1

d   vitamin B_2

e   niacin

f   vitamin C

g   zinc

h   selenium

i   iron.

Questions 31–33 refer to conditions that are caused by a deficiency in a particular mineral or vitamin. Choose the most appropriate answer from the options listed. Each option may be used once, more than once or not at all.

31 Pellagra

32 Beriberi

33 Scurvy

34 Which of the following statements regarding protein-energy malnutrition are *true*?

   a   Protein-energy malnutrition is a problem of the developing world only.

   b   Marasmus is caused primarily by a low-calorific diet.

   c   Marasmus is characterised by the presence of oedema in the infant.

   d   Kwashiorkor tends to occur at the time when the child is weaned from breast milk.

   e   Children with kwashiorkor are usually ravenous and have a very good appetite.

35 Late walker, obese with insatiable appetite and hyperphagia, poor suck as infant and low intelligence quotient. Which of the following syndromes best describes this child?

   a   Angelman's syndrome

   b   Down's syndrome

   c Prader–Willi's syndrome

   d Edwards's syndrome

   e Rubella syndrome

Bibliography

Barr DGD, Crofton PM, Goel KM. Disorders of bones, joints and connective tissue. In: Campbell AGM, McIntosh N, editors. *Forfar and Arneil's Textbook of Pediatrics*. 5th ed. New York, NY: Churchill Livingstone; 1998. pp. 1544–615.

Brown JK, Minns RA. Disorders of the central nervous system: surgical paediatrics. In: Campbell AGM, McIntosh N, editors. *Forfar and Arneil's Textbook of Pediatrics*. 5th ed. New York, NY: Churchill Livingstone; 1998. pp. 641–846.

Gardner-Medwin JM, Dolezalova P, Cummins C, *et al.* Incidence of Henoch-Schönlein purpura, Kawasaki disease, and rare vasculitides in children of different ethnic origins. *Lancet*. 2002 Oct 19; **360**(9341): 1197–202.

Gunay-Aygun M, Schwartz S, Heeger S, *et al.* The changing purpose of Prader-Willi syndrome clinical diagnostic criteria and proposed revised criteria. *Pediatrics*. 2001 Nov; **108**(5): E92.

Hendricks WM. Pellagra and pellagralike dermatoses: etiology, differential diagnosis, dermatopathology, and treatment. *Semin Dermatol*. 1991 Dec; **10**(4): 282–92.

Jauhola O, Ronkainen J, Koskimies O, *et al.* Outcome of Henoch-Schönlein purpura 8 years after treatment with a placebo or prednisone at disease onset. *Pediatr Nephrol*. 2012 Jun; **27**(6): 933–9.

Mrusek S, Krüger M, Greiner P, *et al.* Henoch-Schönlein purpura. *Lancet*. 2004 Apr 3; **363**(9415): 1116.

Ngan V. *Acrodermatitis Enteropathica*. DermNet NZ; updated 2004. Available at: http://dermnetnz.org/systemic/acrodermatitis-enteropathica.html (accessed 29 May 2013).

Saulsbury FT. Clinical update: Henoch-Schönlein purpura. *Lancet*. 2007 Mar 24; **369**(9566): 976–8.

Tizard EJ. Henoch-Schönlein purpura. *Arch Dis Child*. 1999 Apr; **80**(4): 380–3.

Tizard EJ, Hamilton-Ayres MJJ. Henoch Schönlein purpura. *Arch Dis Child Pract Ed*. 2008 Feb; **93**(1): 1–8.

Watanabe T. Henoch-Schönlein purpura following influenza vaccinations during the pandemic of influenza A (H1N1). *Pediatr Nephrol.* 2011 May; **26**(5): 795–8. Epub 2010 Dec 1.

Weaver LT. Nutrition. In: Campbell AGM, McIntosh N, editors. *Forfar and Arneil's Textbook of Pediatrics.* 5th ed. New York, NY: Churchill Livingstone; 1998. pp. 1179–230.

Gastro-oesophageal reflux disease

Four-month-old Alex is next on the list. On reading his notes you see that he developed 'acid reflux' in the second month of his life. Repeated visits to the health visitor and GP ensued over the following 8 weeks. It appears that he spits up lots of his milk and is generally inconsolable for half an hour after feeding. Mum reports refusal of breast and formula milk as if he is in pain during feeding. After failed reassurances, your colleague prescribed an alginate-containing preparation, to be taken mixed with his feeds. Notes from the health visitor confirm healthy growth along the 50th centile. Today mum would like you to prescribe a proton pump inhibitor (PPI) for Alex. She has read about Alex's problems and tells you that all his symptoms are suggestive of gastro-oesophageal reflux disease (GERD). She would like to try Alex on a PPI, as she has read that they are extremely effective for acid reflux. She is troubled by Alex being in so much pain and feels nobody is taking his problem seriously.

Which of the following statements regarding GERD are *true*?

a   Alex must have an endoscopy before a prescription of a PPI is considered, as his symptoms are indicative of underlying pathology.

b   PPIs have been shown to be very effective in treating GERD in infants under the age of 1 year.

c   Use of gastric acidity inhibitors, such as PPIs, have been linked with increased risk of community-acquired pneumonia in children.

d   Prone positioning of the infant is associated with a reduced risk of acid reflux in the infant.

e   Infants under the age of 10 weeks require higher doses of PPIs than older children because of rapid clearance of the drug.

Answer: c and d

GERD refers to the involuntary reflux of stomach contents into the oesophagus, causing irritation and damage. Whereas an adult may complain of heartburn, chest pain or burning, bloating, nausea and an acidic taste in the mouth, the presentation in children and infants is less likely to be so obvious. In most cases the reflux is minor and is an annoyance. It causes irritation in the child and may be responsible for unexplained bouts of vomiting. When reflux is suspected in a child, the important differentiation to be made is whether it is simple physiological reflux that is likely to self-resolve or whether complications of GERD are developing. Whereas the former can be managed by reassurance and conservative measures, the latter is likely to require treatment. Figure 3 may be useful in helping differentiate between mild and severe disease.

   GERD has been linked with asthma, bronchitis and pneumonia. Sandifer's syndrome is a rare but interesting presentation of GERD. The child presents with spastic torticollis and dystonic movements thought to be due to acid reflux. This is often mistaken for seizures and the child is usually seen in neurology clinics prior to a gastrointestinal cause being considered. Investigations tend to reveal evidence of severe GERD and medical or surgical treatment of the reflux resolves the 'neurological' manifestations.

   The large majority of cases encountered in primary care will be of mild, non-chronic reflux. These are presumably caused by transient, non-swallowing-related relaxation of the lower oesophageal sphincter coupled with delayed gastric emptying and gut dysmotility. The peak age of incidence

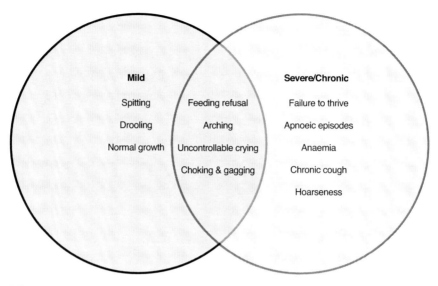

FIGURE 3

is at 4 months of age and the large majority of these infants will be symptom free by the end of the second year of their life. Spontaneous resolution is less likely if reflux symptoms develop after the age of 3 years. Alex is likely to have mild reflux, as he does not exhibit any features of severe disease as listed earlier. In this case it is important to explore the mother's concerns and expectations. Often it is the crying that causes the most parental distress, rather than the spitting or posseting of feeds. The parents' understanding of normal child behaviour should be explored. If parental concern over normal childhood behaviour is suspected, it is important to explain this and resist the need to write out a prescription. With short consultation times it is occasionally easier to write out a prescription than to delve into the details of the problem. Knowing when and what to prescribe is an important skill of medicine, but a finer practitioner of the art knows when not to prescribe. We must resist our own instinct of 'over-medicalising' every problem. Children spit and cry; a shorter oesophagus and distension of a non-compliant abdomen and oesophagus post feed is more likely to be responsible than an acidic reflux. When mild disease is suspected it may be beneficial to avoid the term 'acid reflux', as this implies an abnormality that needs to be corrected by 'anti-reflux' measures. Parents should be made aware that recent booms in the use of PPIs in infants under the age of 1 year are not backed by evidence. Moreover, PPIs are not licensed for use in the UK for children under the age of 1 year. Use of PPIs and other gastric acidity inhibitors has been linked with gastrointestinal and respiratory infections, vitamin deficiencies, food allergy, interstitial nephritis and liver function test abnormalities. Parents should be reassured that crying, arching or turning away from the bottle or breast is part of normal infant behaviour. It is important not to underestimate the importance of reassurance and explanation and will generally receive more appreciation that just writing up a script. Crying will usually respond to patting, rocking or taking the child for a car ride. One interesting study looked at the efficacy of conservative measures in the management of GERD in infants (Orenstein and McGowan, 2008). Bottle-fed infants were provided with semi-elemental formula feeds thickened with dry rice cereal whereas breastfeeding mothers were advised to avoid cow's milk and soy products in their diet. Parents were advised to avoid keeping their child seated or supine, particularly after feeds, and to avoid infant exposure to tobacco smoke. This study found that conservative measures in the primary care setting improved GERD symptoms in 78% of infants, normalising in 24%. Although the study did not show which one of the individual measures produced the most effect, it would be reasonable to suggest all three to parents. Semi-elemental feeds and allergen avoidance in breastfeeding mothers need only be temporary measures, as gradual introduction of cow's milk and other antigens into the diet can be encouraged after the initial difficult period is over. Although it has been associated with sudden infant death syndrome, the flat prone position is the most desirable position for children with GERD. Smoking should be avoided, as passive exposure in children has been associated with oesophagitis and reduction in the tone of the lower oesophagus with delayed gastric transit time, thereby increasing acid reflux.

Cases of severe GERD will require further assessment and management. A prokinetic agent, such as domperidone, used in combination with an H_2-receptor antagonist, such as ranitidine, is common practice in the pharmacological management of GERD in children. PPIs have been shown to be very effective in the management of GERD and its complications. Omeprazole is licensed for use in children over the age of 1 year who have severe ulcerating oesophagitis. It is available in a multiple-unit pellet system that can be administered after mixing in fruit juice or yogurt. Surgical treatment, such as fundoplication and the placement of a percutaneous gastrojejunostomy tube, is reserved for the most severe and refractory cases.

Examination practice: causative agents

Options for questions 36–38:

a   *Coxiella burnetii*

b   Measles virus

c   aspirin

d   21-hydroxylase deficiency

e   trisomy 18

f   22q11 chromosome deletion

g   *Borrelia burgdorferi*

h   prenatal lithium use

i   trisomy 21.

Choose the appropriate causative agent for questions 36–38 from the list of options provided. Each option may be used once, more than once or not at all.

36 DiGeorge's syndrome

37 Lyme disease

38 Congenital adrenal hyperplasia (CAH)

39 Which of the following statements regarding *Helicobacter pylori* in children is/are *false*?

    a   Children with *H. pylori* infection present frequently with vague symptoms related to the gastrointestinal tract.

    b   All children with functional abdominal pain should be tested for *H. pylori* infection.

    c   It would be reasonable to test a child for *H. pylori* who is suffering from iron-deficiency anaemia where another cause has not been found.

    d   Serological tests are the gold standard for *H. pylori* detection and diagnosis in children.

    e   Endoscopy, for confirmation of infection, should not be carried out on a child until a positive serological test has been demonstrated.

40 Which of the following is not a recognised complication of nephrotic syndrome in children?

a   Bacterial peritonitis
b   Hypoparathyroidism
c   Myocardial infarction
d   Renal failure
e   Pulmonary embolus

Bibliography

Campbell AGM. Infections. In: Campbell AGM, McIntosh N, editors. *Forfar and Arneil's Textbook of Pediatrics*. 5th ed. New York, NY: Churchill Livingstone; 1998. pp. 1273–543.

Canani RB, Cirillo P, Roggero P, *et al.* Therapy with gastric acidity inhibitors increases the risk of acute gastroenteritis and community-acquired pneumonia in children. *Pediatrics*. 2006 May; **117**(5): e817–20.

Crowley E, Bourke B, Hussey S. How to use *Helicobacter pylori* testing in paediatric practice. *Arch Dis Child Educ Pract Ed*. 2013 Feb; **98**(1): 18–25. Epub 2012 Oct 23.

Davies EG. Immunodeficiency. In: Campbell AGM, McIntosh N, editors. *Forfar and Arneil's Textbook of Pediatrics*. 5th ed. New York, NY: Churchill Livingstone; 1998. pp. 1231–72.

Del Rosario JF, Orenstein SR. Gastrooesophageal reflux. In: David TJ, editor. *Recent Advances in Paediatrics Number 17*. London: Churchill Livingstone; 1999. pp. 161–72.

Eddy AA, Symons JM. Nephrotic syndrome in childhood. *Lancet*. 2003 Aug 23; **362**(9384): 629–39.

Hassall E. Over-prescription of acid suppressing medications in infants: how it came about, why it's wrong and what to do about it. *J Paediatr*. 2012 Feb; **160**(2): 193–8. Epub 2011 Oct 22.

Higginbotham TW. Effectiveness and safety of proton pump inhibitors in infantile gastroesophageal reflux disease. *Ann Pharmacother*. 2010 Mar; **44**(3): 572–6. Epub 2010 Feb 2.

Kelnar CJH. Endocrine gland disorders and disorders of growth and puberty. In: Campbell AGM, McIntosh N, editors. *Forfar and Arneil's Textbook of Pediatrics*. 5th ed. New York, NY: Churchill Livingstone; 1998. pp. 1273–543.

Lehwald N, Krausch M, Franke C, *et al.* Sandifer syndrome: a multidisciplinary diagnostic and therapeutic challenge. *Eur J Pediatr Surg.* 2007 Jun; **17**(3): 203–6.

Litalien C, Théorêt Y, Faure C. Pharmacokinetics of proton pump inhibitors in children. *Clin Pharmacokinet.* 2005; **44**(5): 441–66.

Merke DP, Bornstein SR. Congenital adrenal hyperplasia. *Lancet.* 2005 Jun 18–24; **365**(9477): 2125–36.

Orenstein SR, McGowan JD. Efficacy of conservative therapy as taught in the primary care setting for symptoms suggesting infant gastroesophageal reflux. *J Pediatr.* 2008 Mar; **152**(3): 310–14.

Zhang W, Kukulka M, Witt G, *et al.* Age-dependent pharmacokinetics of lansoprazole in neonates and infants. *Paediatr Drugs.* 2008; **10**(4): 265–74.

Attention deficit hyperactivity disorder

The last patient on your list is 6-year-old Max. His electronic notes indicate that he is a new patient, as he has not been previously seen in the surgery. On calling him from the waiting room you realise he is not there and mum is here alone on his behalf. She enters clutching some empty bottles and paperwork. She tells you that she is here to get a repeat prescription for Max. Max and his family have recently moved to your area from New York. Six months ago Max's paediatrician in the United States diagnosed Max with attention deficit hyperactivity disorder (ADHD). Max's mum shows you the letter from her doctor that confirms the diagnosis. The drugs she wants you to prescribe are as follows:

- *atomoxetine 80 mg, to be taken once a day*
- *melatonin 10 mg, to be taken before bedtime.*

Having been busy with the process of moving, mum failed to realise that Max's medication had completely run out. He is at school today and if he misses his medication his behaviour is severely affected, having a detrimental effect on his studies. She would like you to issue the script today so that there is no break in his treatment.

Which of the following statements is/are *false*?

a Diagnostic criteria for ADHD may differ in the UK when compared with the United States.

b Premature birth is a recognised risk factor for ADHD.

c Atomoxetine is a stimulant medication and hence should not be used in children under the age of 12 years.

d Stimulant medications have been shown to increase appetite and weight, necessitating careful weight monitoring in children taking them.

e Methylphenidate has been shown to increase motivation and interest in healthy subjects by increasing dopamine levels in the brain.

Answer: c and d

Few paediatric conditions have generated controversial debate among the medical and lay community as much as ADHD. The debate among the medical community regarding ADHD has generally been healthy and useful. However, the Gillberg affair (Gornall, 2007) showed how matters had got out of hand, leading to accusations of fraud and the destruction of valuable scientific data. Accusations and counter-accusations between the two camps of those who are strongly in favour of diagnosing ADHD (at a perceived low threshold) and those who believe physicians are prescribing medication under the influence of pharmaceutical companies has left many parents and non-specialised doctors confused. The case outlined here aims to highlight this controversy and its practical implications in the day-to-day work encountered by GPs.

The very beginnings of the controversy may very well be traced to the exact definition of what we are discussing. Terms such as hyperactivity, over-activity, inattention, impulsivity and hyperkinetic disorder (HKD) may all be mentioned when discussing ADHD and they may not be referring to the same problem. Historically, there has been a difference in approach between the United States and Europe when defining the problem. Physicians in the United States use the American Psychiatric Association's *Diagnostic and Statistical Manual of Mental Disorders* (4th edition; DSM-IV) criteria for the diagnosis of ADHD. This requires the presence of a set of symptoms of inattention *and/or* hyperactivity-impulsivity for at least 6 months. The symptoms should be severe and persistent enough to affect the child's social, school or intellectual functioning in more than one setting (home, school, work). This definition allows for three subtypes of ADHD: (1) inattentive ADHD, (2) hyperactive-impulsive ADHD and (3) a mixed type. In Europe the World Health Organization's International Classification of Diseases and Related Health Problems (10th edition; ICD-10) has been used to diagnose HKD. The diagnostic criteria for HKD are stricter, as there are no subsets like in the DSM-IV definition. The ICD-10 criteria requires at least six inattentive, three hyperactive and one impulsive symptom present all together for at least 6 months with the aforementioned effect on child functioning in more than one setting. Both require the onset of symptoms to be before the age of 7 years. Using the DSM-IV criteria the prevalence of ADHD is around 8%. The prevalence is 1% or lower using the ICD-10 criteria. The implications are immediately apparent with this discrepancy in the way that the condition may be defined, as it will result in huge differences in the proportion of young children who will be labelled with the condition. HKD correlates with a more severe form of mixed-type ADHD. However, worryingly, ADHD seems to be becoming the umbrella term to describe all types of ADHD and HKD, even when the stricter diagnostic criteria are being applied. There is a risk of the term 'HKD' being dropped from future discourse on the subject. This is a worrying trend, as it lumps a whole range of varying childhood behaviour under one term, opening the possibility of more children being exposed to medication at a critical time of brain development.

The subjective nature of the diagnostic criteria has also raised concerns. The clinician is largely dependent on parent and teacher reporting of symptoms to make the diagnosis and monitor the effects of treatment. Studies have shown correlation between parent and teacher reporting of improvement in symptoms in children with ADHD taking stimulant medication (Faraone, *et al.*, 2005). The same study, however, showed a lack of correlation when there were concerns of worsening or lack of improvement in symptoms. The conclusion was, thus, when given a report of no improvement from one setting, clinicians cannot be certain about clinical status in the other setting. Also, there does not seem to be an agreement about when the criteria described by DSM-IV and ICD-10 represent ADHD and when they are indicative of developmentally healthy levels of inattention, hyperactivity and impulsivity.

Once other conditions (e.g. learning disorders, oppositional defiant disorder, bipolar disorder, conduct disorder, depression) have been ruled out and a diagnosis of ADHD/HKD has been agreed upon, then consideration must be given to the most controversial aspect of ADHD management: medication. Why does ADHD need to be treated anyway? Studies have shown ADHD to be linked with problems at school and in later work life, antisocial behaviour, family problems and traffic misdemeanours. Children with ADHD are considered at greater risk of developing other psychiatric disorders and substance abuse problems in later life. By using the DSM-IV criteria for diagnosis, the majority of studies make it difficult to elucidate whether all children with a diagnosis of ADHD are at risk of these problems or whether it is restricted to those suffering from the more severe form. This would certainly allow medication to be more targeted to the appropriate children. Studies have consistently shown that pharmacological treatment of ADHD is increasing. However, the same studies have shown that the levels of treatment are still below the quoted prevalence of the condition. In the UK the number of pharmacologically treated children had risen to 0.3 per 100 children in the late 1990s. In the United States the number was as high as 3.4 per 100 children and these numbers continue to rise. Whether one is in the 'ADHD is over-treated' camp or the 'ADHD is under-treated' camp will depend upon the prevalence figures one believes (1% for HKD vs. 8% for ADHD). Studies have demonstrated unnecessary medication of children who may not be suffering from the condition (Angold, *et al.*, 2000). Although regrettable, unnecessary intervention in medicine is not peculiar to ADHD. However, it evokes an emotive response in its detractors. It certainly should not be a reason to accuse well-meaning physicians of fraud and negligence.

The most commonly used medications in the management of ADHD are the central nervous system (CNS) stimulants methylphenidate and dexamfetamine and the noradrenaline reuptake inhibitor atomoxetine. Other drugs that are used less commonly include tricyclic antidepressants, monoamine oxidase inhibitors, α_2-agonists such as clonidine, bupropion and modafinil. CNS stimulants have been used in the management of ADHD for over 4 decades now and their effectiveness is well documented. However, considering the duration of their use, it is surprising that their effects have not been well followed in a detailed manner over many years and into adulthood. Drugs should be started by a specialist with an interest in the management of ADHD in children. Follow-up may involve a shared care protocol with the GP. Methylphenidate is licensed for use in children over the age of 6 years. It is prescribed in either an immediate-release or a sustained-release preparation. The former requires dosages to be given at school, which may be attached with some stigma to the child. Sustained-release preparations allow once-daily dosing, hence preventing this problem. A common side effect of CNS stimulants is a lack of appetite, resulting in poor growth. Therefore, weight and height needs to be monitored every 6 months and the input of a dietitian may be needed if there are any signs of faltering growth. Taking the medication after breakfast is also a useful tip. CNS stimulants may also increase blood pressure and cause tachycardia, necessitating 6-monthly blood pressure and pulse reviews. Methylphenidate is associated with an increase in tic frequency. Medication may be changed if this is a cause of huge distress. Insomnia is another troublesome side effect of the CNS stimulants but may also be due to the ADHD itself. It is occasionally managed with medications such as melatonin and clonidine. Other side effects include lowering of the seizure threshold, psychosis and liver damage. Atomoxetine is a non-CNS stimulant option in the management of ADHD. Maximal effect can take 8 weeks and it may be a useful alternative if troublesome tics develop on methylphenidate. Somnolence is a troublesome side effect of the drug and may be counteracted by giving the drug in the evening. It may also increase pulse rate and blood pressure, and there have been reports of hepatic toxicity and increased suicidal ideation while taking the drug. National Institute for Health and Care Excellence guidelines suggest choosing the cheapest preparation if more than one is appropriate to use in the child.

How one proceeds with the parent in this case will depend on the physician's level of comfort with the diagnostic capabilities of their transatlantic colleague. The diagnosis is almost certainly to have been made using the DSM-IV criteria but the degree of impairment is not apparent in the diagnosis. Not prescribing the medication is likely to upset and antagonise the parent, as the parents are the ones facing the brunt of the disruptive behaviour. It would be appropriate to explain the differences in the diagnostic criteria and the need for confirmation by a child psychiatrist in the UK. A short supply of medication may be prescribed until a suitable assessment can be arranged.

Examination practice: skeletal deformities

Options for questions 41–43:

a   Marfan's syndrome

b   funnel chest

c   pes planus

d   Blount's disease

e   genu valgum

f   Apert's syndrome

g   pectus carinatum

h   Pierre Robin syndrome

i   talipes equinovarus.

Questions 41–43 refer to children presenting with skeletal deformities. Choose the most appropriate diagnosis for each scenario. Each option may be used once, more than once or not at all.

41 Mum brings in 18-month-old Jacob. He has recently started walking. Mum is worried that his left foot seems abnormal on walking. You observe an unbothered Jacob as he hunts for toys in your room. You note a slightly pronated left foot with a flattened arch. Similar features are seen in the right foot but to a lesser extent.

42 Three-month-old Emma has a prominent sternum. Viewed laterally the anteroposterior diameter of the chest is increased. No other physical abnormalities are elicited.

43 A 4-year-old boy presents with progressively worsening bowing of the legs. A bony prominence is felt on the medial aspects of both knees.

44 Which of the following factors is/are associated with an increased prevalence of autism?

   a   A sibling with autism

   b   Maternal use of carbamazepine in pregnancy

   c   Fragile X syndrome

   d   Gestational age of greater than 35 weeks

   e   Down's syndrome

45 Which of the following syndromes represents an association between glomerulonephritis and sensorineural deafness?

a Waardenburg's syndrome

b Usher's syndrome

c Alport's syndrome

d Refsum's syndrome

e Klippel–Feil's syndrome

Bibliography

Angold A, Erkanli A, Egger HL, *et al.* Stimulant treatment for children: a community perspective. *J Am Acad Child Adolesc Psychiatry.* 2000 Aug; **39**(8): 975–84; discussion 984–94.

Barr DGD, Crofton PM, Goel KM. Disorders of bone, joints and connective tissue. In: Campbell AGM, McIntosh N, editors. *Forfar and Arneil's Textbook of Pediatrics.* 5th ed. New York, NY: Churchill Livingstone; 1998. pp. 1544–615.

Biederman J, Faraone SV. Attention-deficit hyperactivity disorder. *Lancet.* 2005 Jul 16–22; **366**(9481): 237–48.

Cowan DL, Kerr AIG. Disorders of the ear, nose and throat. In: Campbell AGM, McIntosh N, editors. *Forfar and Arneil's Textbook of Pediatrics.* 5th ed. New York, NY: Churchill Livingstone; 1998. pp. 1679–88.

Faraone SV, Biederman J, Zimmerman B. Correspondence of parent and teacher reports in medication trials. *Eur Child Adolesc Psychiatry.* 2005 Feb; **14**(1): 20–7.

Gornall J. Hyperactivity in children: the Gillberg affair. *BMJ.* 2007 Aug 25; **335**(7616): 370–3.

Guevara JP, Stein MT. Evidence based management of attention deficit hyperactivity disorder. *BMJ.* 2001 Nov 24; **323**(7323): 1232–5.

Harpin VA. Medication options when treating children and adolescents with ADHD: interpreting the NICE guidance 2006. *Arch Dis Child Educ Pract Ed.* 2008 Apr; **93**(2): 58–65.

Hoare P, Will D, Wrate R. Psychiatric disorders. In: Campbell AGM, McIntosh N, editors. *Forfar and Arneil's Textbook of Pediatrics.* 5th ed. New York, NY: Churchill Livingstone; 1998. pp. 1727–67.

National Institute for Health and Clinical Excellence. *Attention Deficit*

Hyperactivity Disorder: NICE clinical guideline 72. London: NICE; 2008. www.nice.org.uk/CG72

National Institute for Health and Clinical Excellence. *Autism Diagnosis in Children and Young People: NICE clinical guideline 128.* London: NICE; 2011. www.nice.org.uk/CG128

Rappley MD. Clinical practice: attention deficit-hyperactivity disorder. *N Engl J Med.* 2005 Jan 13; **352**(2): 165–73.

Rull G. *Blount's Disease.* Leeds: Patient.co.uk, Egton Medical Information Systems Limited; 2010. Available at: www.patient.co.uk/doctor/Blount's-Disease.htm (accessed 29 May 2013).

Volkow ND, Wang GJ, Fowler JS, *et al.* Evidence that methylphenidate enhances the saliency of a mathematical task by increasing dopamine in the human brain. *Am J Psychiatry.* 2004 Jul; **161**(7): 1173–80.

Skull deformities

The next patient is 4-month-old Emily. You note numerous entries in her notes as mum attended on almost a daily basis for the first 2 months of Emily's life. This was understandable, as she lost her first child to sudden infant death syndrome (SIDS) when he was only 4 weeks old. As expected, most visits for Emily had been for minor problems and mostly only reassurance was required, which was duly given. Today mum tells you that she is worried about the way Emily's head looks. You note flattening of the occiput on the right side with slight ipsilateral forehead prominence. The right ear also seems to be marginally displaced anteriorly when compared with the left ear. One of the health visitors had mentioned to mum that this may be related to abnormal brain development later in life and that she should get it checked out by the doctor. Mum does not think Emily was born with an abnormally shaped head and feels it has developed over the last 2 months. On examination and further questioning you find out that Emily coos appropriately when engaged verbally, can hold her head up steadily and will occasionally reach for toys. No other abnormalities of the skull or face are present. She was born at term and delivered by ventouse. She had a mild cephalohaematoma, which had resolved by the routine 6-week check.

Which of the following statements is/are *true*?

a Plagiocephaly is associated with an increased risk of SIDS.

b Displacement of the ear anteriorly is suggestive of premature lambdoid suture fusion.

c Emily is likely to need surgical intervention to improve skull shape and reduce the risk of developing raised intracranial pressure.

d Maintenance in a supine position, such as that achieved in a car seat, should be encouraged to help achievement of normal skull shape.

e Skull helmets are expensive and have little evidence for their effectiveness in most infants with plagiocephaly.

Answer: e

The highly malleable, soft infantile skull is prone to asymmetrical moulding and misshapenness. External pressures after birth or in utero and intrapartum constraints may give rise to various skull shapes. These are commonly referred to as benign positional skull deformities and are different from the potentially more serious deformities caused by early fusion of one or more of the skull sutures, referred to as craniosynostosis. Attempts at classifying the non-synostotic skull deformities (Wilbrand, *et al.*, 2012) have defined three clinical groups:

1 positional plagiocephaly

2 positional brachycephaly

3 combined positional plagiocephaly and brachycephaly.

Examination of the head from above allows the examiner to appreciate the nature of the abnormality. The typical plagioacephalic head is described as a parallelogram due to unilateral flattening of the occiput with ipsilateral parietal and frontal bossing. However, since the frontal bossing is never as significant as the occipital flattening, the shape of the head from above may appear more trapezoidal. In *positional plagiocephaly*, the ear on the flattened side is displaced anteriorly and the eye may appear more open because of forward movement of the zygoma. This is caused by the infant displaying a preference of keeping his or her head tilted to one side. This may be due to something simple, such as the positioning of the cot in the room, encouraging the child to keep the head turned in the direction of visual and auditory stimulation. However, positional plagiocephaly may also develop due to torticollis, which may be congenital (due to in utero pressures) or acquired (due to persistent unidirectional head positioning and limited neck movement). In either case the sternocleidomastoid muscle is shortened and contracted on one side while lack of use may result in atrophy of the muscle on the opposite side. Clinically it will manifest with the infant unable to turn his or her head away from the affected side while being turned and trying to maintain gaze at an object of interest such as his or her parent. *Positional brachycephaly* is when the occipital flattening is symmetrical, resulting in the head appearing disproportionately wider when viewed from the front. This will occur in the child left mostly on his or her back with little respite from the external pressure on the posterior part of the growing skull. *Combined positional plagiocephaly and brachycephaly* may also be referred to as asymmetrical brachycephaly (Rogers, 2011a), as although there is bilateral occipital flattening, it is more pronounced on one side. Scaphocephaly is a type of plagiocephaly in which the side of the head is flattened with elongation of the skull anteriorly and posteriorly resulting in a long, thin head. This is seen in infants who lie on their sides for prolonged periods, as may be the case in premature infants in intensive care units. It is thought that the 'Back to Sleep' campaign in the United States, encouraging parents to lay their children on their backs to prevent the risk of SIDS, has contributed to the increased risk of positional skull deformities.

For a GP performing routine child health checks, it is important to be able to differentiate the aforementioned deformities from craniosynostosis. The routine 6- to 8-week check involves examination of the skull sutures. The coronal, saggital and lambdoidal sutures should be felt for ridging, which represents early fusion of the sutures. This may be normal, it may represent isolated congenital craniosynostosis or it may be part of a syndrome (e.g. Apert's syndrome, Crouzon's syndrome). If ridging is felt then the skull should be examined for deformities. Unilateral coronal craniosynostosis causes anterior plagiocephaly with flattening of the ipsilateral forehead (as opposed to bossing seen in positional plagiocephaly). Lambdoidal craniosynostosis is difficult to differentiate from positional plagiocephaly but is thankfully much less common. Two distinguishing features present in lambdoidal cranosynostosis include inferior and posterior displacement of the ear on the affected side (as opposed to anterior displacement as seen in positional plagiocephaly) and a bony prominence in the mastoid area. Asymmetrical occipital flattening is present in both. Saggital craniosyn-ostosis may mimic scaphocephaly with the former rarely exhibiting any facial asymmetry. If craniosynostosis is suspected, a referral to a paediatric craniofacial surgeon with expertise in assessment and management should be done, as surgery is usually needed to correct the abnormal skull shape.

Non-synostotic skull deformities may be managed conservatively. Advice should be given on the need for 'tummy time' when the infant is placed prone to reduce pressure on the growing skull. This can be done during the day under supervision. Prolonged supine positioning in car seats should be avoided. If necessary, cot positioning should be altered and the child should be put to sleep on alternating occiputs. If torticollis is found, then massage of the neck muscles may be encouraged to help loosen the contracture in the muscle. The sternocleidomastoid and trapezius muscles need to be stretched and strengthened through manual mobilisation exercises. The neck is rotated to encourage the chin and ear to touch the ipsilateral shoulder in separate movements. Each position is held for approximately 10 seconds. This can be done during routine nappy changes. Stretching exercises can be incorporated into play, with one parent sitting with the child while the other encourages neck movements by getting the child to concentrate on a toy or other object of interest while moving side to side in front of the child. The movements need to be large enough to result in the child rotating his or her neck. These measures will usually suffice in correcting the skull abnormality if persevered with for 2–3 months.

Intentional modification of the infant skull shape has been practised by many cultures for many centuries (Obladen, 2012). This may have been for aesthetic reasons or for identification with a particular social status. It is therefore not surprising that parents often ask about the use of skull-moulding helmets in the management of positional plagiocephaly. Also known as cranial banding, this involves a custom-made, foam-lined rigid helmet that is worn by the infant at all times, except when washing. They work by allowing increased growth in the flattened area by cutting out the foam around it. They require regular checking to ensure good skin health at points of contact. They generally have a very good safety record. They are usually worn between 6 and 12 months of age. However, evidence for their effectiveness is scant, particularly when compared against conservative measures discussed earlier. They are also very expensive (£2000–£3000). Therefore, they are generally not available on the National Health Service.

Most positional deformities, with time, will become less apparent as the infant skull enlarges and grows more hair. Since the deformities are more visible when viewed from above, as the child grows in height they will become less of a concern. One study followed 129 children up to 4 years of age and found that overall head shape measurements, parental concerns and developmental delays observed in infancy had dramatically improved when re-measured at 3 and 4 years of age (Hutchison, *et al.*, 2010). Indications for specialist referral of children with positional skull deformities include failure to correct or progression of deformity despite conservative measures, torticollis not responding to stretching exercises or when the diagnosis is in doubt.

Examination practice: appropriate management

Options for questions 46–48:

a   eye test

b   simple analgesia

c   antihypertensive

d   magnetic resonance imaging of the brain

e   pizotifen

f   100% oxygen

g   oral contraceptive pill

h   blood pressure recording.

For questions 46–48 choose the most appropriate management option from the list provided. Each option may be used once, more than once or not at all.

46 A 12-year-old girl presents with a 1-year history of periodic, pulsating, unilateral headache with no obvious trigger. The headache is preceded by flashes of light in the ipsilateral eye and is accompanied by nausea. The headache disappears with a combination of simple analgesia and lying down. Mum suffers from similar attacks. The frequency of headaches is now beginning to affect school. Neurological examination is normal.

47 A 6-year-old boy presents with mum who reports a 3-month history of intermittent frontal headache that occasionally extends to behind the eyes. It is usually present in the latter part of the day and settles with simple analgesia or having a rest. The child is otherwise well.

48 A 15-year-old boy presents to casualty with a third episode of intense right-sided headache that came on suddenly. He appears agitated and restless and you find it difficult to perform an adequate neurological examination. His ipsilateral eye is red and watery and appears swollen. The last two episodes, which occurred in the last 2 weeks, lasted about an hour each.

49 Which of the following statements regarding Hodgkin's lymphoma are *true*?

    a   Lower socio-economic groups are associated with a greater risk of developing Hodgkin's disease.

b Epstein–Barr virus infection has been implicated strongly in the development of Hodgkin's lymphoma.

c Reed–Sternberg cells are pathognomonic of Hodgkin's lymphoma.

d The presence of B symptoms is associated with a worse prognosis.

e St Jude staging system is used to stage Hodgkin's lymphoma.

50 Deficiency of factor IX results in which inherited condition?

a Christmas disease

b Von Willebrand's disease

c Haemophilia A

d Idiopathic thrombocytopaenic purpura

e Bernard–Soulier's syndrome

Bibliography

Brown JK, Minns RA. Disorders of the central nervous system. In: Campbell AGM, McIntosh N, editors. *Forfar and Arneil's Textbook of Pediatrics.* 5th ed. New York, NY: Churchill Livingstone; 1998. pp. 641–846.

Eden OB. Oncology and terminal care. In: Campbell AGM, McIntosh N, editors. *Forfar and Arneil's Textbook of Pediatrics.* 5th ed. New York, NY: Churchill Livingstone; 1998. pp. 884–933.

Gil-Gouveia R, Martins IP. Headaches associated with refractive errors: myth or reality? *Headache.* 2002 Apr; **42**(4): 256–62.

Hutchison BL, Stewart AW, Mitchell EA. Deformational plagiocephaly: a follow-up of head shape, parental concern and neurodevelopment at ages 3 and 4 years. *Arch Dis Child.* 2011 Jan; **96**(1): 85–90. Epub 2010 Sep 29.

Jones BM, Hayward R, Evans R, *et al.* Occipital plagiocephaly: an epidemic of craniosynostosis? *BMJ.* 1997 Sep 20; **315**(7110): 693–4.

King DJ. Disorders of the blood and reticuloendothelial system. In: Campbell AGM, McIntosh N, editors. *Forfar and Arneil's Textbook of Pediatrics.* 5th ed. New York, NY: Churchill Livingstone; 1998. pp. 847–83.

Laughlin J, Luerssen TG, Dias MS; Committee on Practice and Ambulatory Medicine, Section on Neurological Surgery. Prevention and management of positional skull deformities in infants. *Pediatrics.* 2011 Dec; **128**(6): 1236–41. Epub 2011 Nov 28.

Majumdar A, Ahmed MA, Benton S. Cluster headache in children: experience from a specialist headache clinic. *Eur J Paediatr Neurol.* 2009 Nov; **13**(6): 524–9. Epub 2008 Dec 23.

Obladen M. In God's image? The tradition of infant head shaping. *J Child Neurol.* 2012 May; **27**(5): 672–80. Epub 2012 Feb 28.

Rogers GF. Deformational plagiocephaly, brachycephaly, and scaphocephaly. Part I: terminology, diagnosis, and etiopathogenesis. *J Craniofac Surg.* 2011a Jan; **22**(1): 9–16.

Rogers GF. Deformational plagiocephaly, brachycephaly, and scaphocephaly. Part II: prevention and treatment. *J Craniofac Surg.* 2011b Jan; **22**(1): 17–23.

Wilbrand JF, Schmidtberg K, Bierther U, *et al.* Clinical classification of infant nonsynostotic cranial deformity. *J Pediatr.* 2012 Dec; **161**(6): 1120–5. Epub 2012 Jun 23.

Bronchiolitis

On a chilly December evening, as you start your emergency night shift, your first patient is a 6-month-old infant. Mum tells you that for the last 2 days Jake has had a runny nose and fever. Today his breathing has been affected. He has also been feeding less than usual, taking to the breast half as much as usual. His older sibling suffers from asthma and mum used his salbutamol inhaler on Jake a few hours ago with little effect. Mum wonders whether a nebuliser is more appropriate. Jake was born at 34 weeks' gestation by spontaneous delivery with no complications. He did not require respiratory support at birth. On examination you find Jake reasonably comfortable at rest, with a respiratory rate of 50 with minimal subcostal recession. Auscultation reveals fine crackles spread all over the chest, with scattered mild wheeze, whereas chest percussion is normal. Pulse oximetry reveals oxygen saturation levels of 94% and his temperature is 38.2°C.

Which of the following statements is/are *false*?

a   Respiratory syncytial virus (RSV) is the most common cause of acute bronchiolitis.

b   The large majority of children will have serological evidence of RSV infection by the age of 3, rendering them immune to any further infections from the virus.

c Jake should be admitted for a chest X-ray, as the combination of low oxygen saturations and fine crackles means that pneumonia needs ruling out.

d Bronchodilators are not routinely recommended in the management of bronchiolitis.

e Prophylactic RSV immunoglobulin may play a protective role in a small group of infants at risk of severe disease.

Answer: b and c

Bronchiolitis is a common infection, usually in the first year of life, associated with significant infant morbidity. RSV is the commonest causative agent, although other viruses have also been implicated. Some, such as adenovirus, are more likely to be associated with serious long-term complications such as obliterative bronchiolitis. Epidemics of the causative agents usually occur between November and March, resulting in spikes in cases of acute bronchiolitis. Although the large majority of children by the age of 3 will have had RSV infection, re-infection is common, as the initial infection appears not to confer protective immunity to the child, a fact that has hindered the development of an effective vaccine.

Clinically, Jake's presentation is typical of how the condition presents. RSV typically infects the nasopharynx at the beginning of the illness, resulting in the prodromal 'runny nose' phase. Direct spread from the nasopharynx and aspiration of the nasopharyngeal secretions is likely to be responsible for the spread of infection from the upper to the lower respiratory tract. This typically occurs over 1–3 days, resulting in worsening respiratory distress, tachypnoea and typical fine crackles with or without wheeze. Most infants will have a fever but this is usually not very high. High temperatures, such as those above 40°C, may represent an alternative source of infection, which should be appropriately investigated for. Reduced feeding is also seen as the dyspnoea worsens. Occasionally, particularly in premature and low birthweight infants, an apnoeic episode may be the presenting feature of bronchiolitis.

The role of investigations is limited, as the diagnosis of bronchiolitis is primarily clinical. However, it is useful to perform pulse oximetry, as this helps gauge the severity of illness. Lower oxygen saturations (≤92%) increase the likelihood of the assessing physician admitting the child into hospital. Oxygen saturations between 92% and 94% require careful assessment of the stage of illness in the child. If the condition is beginning to improve then it may be appropriate for the child to be kept at home. Parents should be made aware of the general course of the condition and be given specific advice about when to seek help. Signs of respiratory distress (tracheal tug, sub- and intercostal recession, cyanosis) should be explained to parents. Other things to look out for would be a reduction of 50% or more in the intake of feeds over the preceding 24 hours, lethargy and apnoeic episodes. The presence of these features suggests severe disease and a paediatric opinion should be sought irrespective of the oxygen saturations. Further investigations in hospital may not be carried out, as they are unlikely to influence the management. Chest radiography is rarely useful and should not be routinely performed. The diagnosis of RSV bronchiolitis may be confirmed by direct viral immunofluorescence on a nasopharyngeal aspirate sample. This may be useful at the start of the RSV season, where isolation of the infant may be desirable to reduce nosocomial infection. However, once the ward is full of children with likely RSV infection it may no longer be performed. Capillary blood gas measurement is usually reserved for children who are clinically worsening and those in whom intensive care therapy is anticipated.

Just as there are very few investigations that may help confirm the disease, there are limited therapeutic options available to alter the course of the condition. Treatment is generally supportive. Many studies have looked at the role of bronchodilators in the treatment of bronchiolitis and have found no convincing evidence of their benefit. They may have a role to play in helping reduce the severity of wheeze in the short term but they certainly have no impact on reducing the duration of stay in hospital or admission to intensive care. Similarly disappointing results have been observed with inhaled bronchodilator therapy. Nevertheless, they are not infrequently used in the child with bronchiolitis, probably because the attending physician feels he or she needs to do something. Other therapeutic options that have been studied include nebulised epinephrine and dexamethasone. Compared with placebo, they too have been found to be ineffective and, therefore, their use is also not recommended. Antivirals, in the form of nebulised ribavarin, and antibiotics are also not recommended for use in infants with bronchiolitis, because of the lack of evidence of their benefit. Measures in hospital that are useful include supplemental oxygen, gentle nasal suction to help keep the nasal passages clear of discharge and supplemental feeding in those severely affected. Hence the purpose of hospital admission is to support the child while he or she recovers from this self-limiting illness. Although not routinely recommended, one study has shown benefit of the leukotriene receptor antagonist montelukast in providing symptomatic relief from the troublesome symptoms of post-infection cough and wheeze (which may persist for weeks to years). It was used in children ranging from 3 to 36 months in age and was shown to increase the number of symptom-free days when started within 7 days of the onset of symptoms and continued for 28 days (Bisgaard and Study Group on Montelukast and Respiratory Syncytial Virus, 2002).

Parents tend to worry that bronchiolitis heralds the onset of asthma. They should be reassured that this is generally not the case and the cough and wheeze associated with bronchiolitis will eventually settle in most cases. However, it is not uncommon to see subsequent wheezing episodes in children who suffered from bronchiolitis when young, particularly in association with viral infections. These can be managed with standard bronchodilator therapy. It is possible that an atopic tendency that predisposes to asthma also predisposes to the development of bronchiolitis, rather than the bronchiolitis being the causative agent in the development of asthma. The RSV immunoglobulin palivizumab can be considered as preventive therapy in a small selective group of infants who are at high risk of developing bronchiolitis. These include infants under the age of 1 year who were born extremely premature or with underlying cardiopulmonary disease or immunodeficiency.

Examination practice: viral illnesses

Options for questions 51–53:

a Coxsackie group A virus

b parvovirus B19

c herpes simplex virus

d human herpes virus 6

e human papillomavirus

f varicella zoster virus

g Epstein–Barr virus

h mumps virus.

From the options above, choose the most likely causative agent in the children presenting with viral illnesses in questions 51–53. Each option may be used once, more than once or not at all.

51 A 14-year-old boy presents with bilaterally enlarged parotid glands and a painful swollen right testicle.

52 A 4-year-old girl presents with a sore throat, low-grade fever and small blisters on her hand, her feet and inside her mouth.

53 A 3-year-old boy develops a high temperature, runny nose and watery eyes. The temperature finally abates on the fourth day and, just as mum thought he was improving, he breaks out in a pinkish rash on his torso that is spreading to his arms and legs. The rash blanches on pressure and disappears after 48 hours.

54 Which of the following statements regarding vaccinations are *true*?

    a Diphtheria, tetanus and pertussis vaccine may be associated with an increased mortality from infections other that diphtheria, tetanus and pertussis in high-mortality areas.

    b The child's response to vaccines may differ depending on the vaccinations and infections they may have had in the past.

    c The measles vaccine has been associated with a reduced mortality from infections other than measles.

    d Vaccination of pregnant mothers with the pertussis vaccine to prevent neonatal infections is not recommended, because of the risk of Arthus's reactions.

e   Vaccinating close household contacts of young infants against pertussis does not reduce the risk of pertussis acquisition by the infant.

55 Which of the following is/are not a live vaccine?

a   Measles

b   Rubella

c   Oral polio

d   Rabies

e   Rotavirus

Bibliography

Amirthalingham G. Strategies to control pertussis in infants. *Arch Dis Child.* 2013 Jul; **98**: 552–5. Epub 2013 May 22.

Bisgaard H; Study Group on Montelukast and Respiratory Syncytial Virus. A randomized trial of montelukast in respiratory syncytial virus postbronchiolitis. *Am J Respir Crit Care Med.* 2003 Feb 1; **167**(3): 379–83. Epub 2002 Oct 3.

Bush A, Thomson AH. Acute bronchiolitis. *BMJ.* 2007 Nov 17; **335**(7628): 1037–41.

Campbell AGM. Infections. In: Campbell AGM, McIntosh N, editors. *Forfar and Arneil's Textbook of Pediatrics.* 5th ed. New York, NY: Churchill Livingstone; 1998. pp. 1273–543.

Domachowske JB, Rosenberg HF. Respiratory syncytial virus infection: immune response, immunopathogenesis, and treatment. *Clin Microbiol Rev.* 1999 Apr; **12**(2): 298–309.

Scottish Intercollegiate Guidelines Network (SIGN). *Bronchiolitis in Children: a national clinical guideline.* Guideline no. 91. Edinburgh: SIGN; 2006. www.sign.ac.uk/pdf/sign91.pdf

Shann F. The non-specific effects of vaccines. *Arch Dis Child.* 2010 Sep; **95**(9): 662–7.

World Health Organization (WHO). *SAGE Working Group on Non-specific Effects of Vaccines (Established March 2013).* Geneva: WHO; 2013. Available at:

www.who.int/immunization/sage/sage_wg_non_specific_effects_vaccines_march2013/en/index.html (accessed 3 September 2013).

Zorc JJ, Hall CB. Bronchiolitis: recent evidence on diagnosis and management. *Pediatrics*. 2010 Feb; **125**(2): 342–9. Epub 2010 Jan 25.

Diabetes

Mum presents with 4-year-old Jodie who has started bedwetting again after a long period of dryness. Mum tells you that this has been happening for the last month. She felt it was due to the stress Jodie may be feeling from starting nursery, as she has had trouble settling in. Jodie's teacher has also noted that she frequently attends the toilet during the 4 hours she is there. Jodie is otherwise a well and active child and has had been reasonably well apart from the usual childhood ailments. Her weight is steady and she has a good appetite. Recently she has started to complain of soreness on passing urine. Mum has noticed mild inflammation around Jodie's genitalia and wondered whether she was suffering from a urinary tract infection. You dip test a sample of urine that mum has brought and find that it is negative for leucocytes and nitrites but positive for urinary glucose.

Which of the following statements is/are *true*?

a   The urine should be sent for microscopy and culture as glycosuria in the context of a well child is likely to represent a urine infection.

b   Diabetes needs ruling out, so Jodie should be given an appointment for a fasting blood glucose test.

c   Diabetes in children under 5 years old can only be confirmed by a glucose tolerance test.

d   The false negative rate of urine glucose testing is low.
e   All newly diagnosed diabetics under the age of 5 should be referred for consideration of islet cell transplantation.

Answer: none of these are true

Prompt diagnosis of type 1 diabetes mellitus (T1DM) in children poses a significant challenge because of the non-specific symptoms with which it may initially present. This is more so the case in younger children. Parents are often aware that something is not right, as the child may complain of vague symptoms of abdominal pain, headaches and tiredness or present with constipation or oral and vaginal thrush, among other conditions. The presence of secondary enuresis should certainly raise suspicion and lead to urine testing. Weight loss coupled with polyuria and polydipsia should also have the alarm bells ringing. Missed and delayed diagnosis can have devastating consequences for the child in the form of diabetic ketoacidosis (DKA). As the vague symptoms continue, the child gets increasingly dehydrated and fatigued and may present in a comatose state. The mortality and morbidity associated with severe DKA is significant and the aim is to identify children at an earlier stage and start appropriate treatment.

Once suspected, the diagnosis of diabetes is not difficult. Historically, it was noted that the urine in diabetes sufferers was sweet. A urine test will confirm the presence of glucose, and should be followed by a single, immediate capillary blood glucose test. Capillary blood sugar levels greater than 11.1 mmol/L are diagnostic of diabetes. No further investigation is required in primary care and the child should be referred to hospital for further assessment. This should be treated as a medical emergency and the child must be seen in secondary care on the same day. At this stage it is appropriate to tell parents what you think the problem is. This is usually fairly distressing news to the parents, as most understand the chronic nature of the condition. The purpose of admission on the same day is to start insulin straight away to prevent the likelihood of developing the aforementioned DKA. On arrival in hospital the diagnosis will be confirmed with blood glucose testing from a venous sample. In primary care, to reduce the risk of a false positive, it is important to wash and dry the child's hands prior to taking the capillary blood glucose measurement to prevent the child's latest sweet snack contributing to a high reading and causing unnecessary distress.

Once the child is referred to secondary care, it is likely the child will not be seen by his or her GP for a while. This is usually because of the comprehensive nature of multidisciplinary input the child and family receive in secondary care. Once diagnosis is confirmed, insulin will be started on the same day. Insulin is usually classified according to the speed of onset, peak and duration of its action. Hence, the various insulins available for use may be rapid-acting analogues (lispro, aspart), fast-acting, intermediate-acting or very long-acting analogues (detemir, glargine) with duration of action ranging from 3 to 24 hours. Rapid-acting analogues will reach peak activity within 2 hours, whereas very long-acting analogues will work steadily in the background over the course of 24 hours without showing any peak activity. As in adults, insulin treatment will need to be individualised in the child for best response. One option may be in the form of a basal-bolus regimen in which insulin detemir or glargine is given, usually at night, to cover background insulin requirements. This is supplemented with rapid- or short-acting insulin at mealtimes. Although this offers a greater deal of flexibility, it does involve more injections, which may be distressing to the child (and parents). The use of a combination of insulins, with varying speeds of onset of action, may reduce the number of injections needed during the day. Another form of insulin therapy, the use of which is gathering momentum in children, is continuous subcutaneous insulin infusion or insulin pump therapy. Insulin pumps work by delivering a preset amount of insulin continuously during the course of the day via a pump and subcutaneously placed infusion set. Further boluses of insulin can be given after eating by pressing a button on the pump. Hence, this system attempts to mimic the pancreas by giving a steady supply of insulin during the day, with postprandial peaks to deal with the sudden peaks in blood sugar levels after eating. It does require regular blood sugar testing during the day and dose adjustment as required. Ideally, a closed-loop system could be developed in which sensors may measure blood sugar levels and automatically adjust the dose of insulin delivered, a true imitation of normal physiology. Although insulin pump therapy sounds ideal for the erratically eating, unpredictably exercising, frequently unwell (with viral infections) young child, further studies are required to determine whether it has a significant impact on quality of life and reducing HbA1c levels.

The role of patient and carer education is of paramount importance to successful management of diabetes. A great deal of anxiety usually accompanies the diagnosis and a specialised multidisciplinary team needs to be at hand to offer support and allay fears. Familiarity with the various devices needs to be learnt and the importance of tight glucose control needs to be explained. It is important that carers are familiar with diabetic ketoacidosis and hypoglycaemia. The importance of tight control early in the condition has been rigorously demonstrated in the Diabetes Control and Complications Trial and the subsequent Epidemiology of Diabetes Interventions and Complications study. The poorer the control, the more likely one is of developing the micro- and macrovascular complications of diabetes. Too tight a control needs to be balanced against the risk of developing hypoglycaemia. The family should have access to a dietitian who is available to give individualised diet advice.

An exciting treatment modality in the management of T1DM, which parents may enquire about, is islet cell transplantation. The fact that the autoimmune destruction of the β-cells of the islets of Langerhan in the pancreas causes diabetes has harboured hope that their replacement should cure the illness. However, things have not been so straightforward. The procedure itself remains expensive and is hampered by the lack of high-quality donor organs for isolation of these cells. Recipients need lifelong immunosuppressive therapy. Hence, it is reserved for patients with very poorly controlled diabetes with recurrent hypoglycaemia and hypoglycaemia unawareness. Unfortunately, the large majority of transplanted patients are likely to need insulin within 5 years. However, it has been shown to improve hypoglycaemia awareness, a benefit that seems to last longer than 5 years. Although not having fulfilled the initial hopes that were attached to islet cell transplantation a decade ago, it may still see rejuvenation as an insulin-sparing treatment with the development of stem cell research and potential limitless supplies of islet cells in the future.

Examination practice: treatment options

Options for questions 56–58:

a mebendazole

b rifampicin

c pyrazinamide

d oestrogen cream

e podophyllotoxin

f clobetasol propionate (0.05%) steroid cream

g oral hydrocortisone

h fluconazole

i none of the above.

Choose the most appropriate treatment option for each of the children presenting in questions 56–58. Each option may be used once, more than once or not at all.

56 The mother of a 2-year-old girl is concerned by the appearance of the girl's genitalia. On examination you note a flat vulva with adhesions extending anteriorly. Mum reports dribbling of urine.

57 A 5-year-old boy is troubled with an intense anal itch. Nothing is obvious on anal examination but you notice that he has damaged nails from compulsive nail biting.

58 A 7-year-old girl presents with a 2-day history of high fever, conjunctivitis and a harsh cough. A reddish blanching rash is noted on the face and upper torso. Inside the mouth you note greyish white Koplik's spots on the buccal mucosa.

59 Which of the following statements regarding type 2 diabetes mellitus (T2DM) in children is/are *true*?

   a T2DM (rather than T1DM) is the more likely diagnosis in the obese child presenting with hyperglycaemia.

   b Prompt differentiation between T1DM and T2DM is the primary objective in a child presenting with diabetic ketoacidosis.

   c Low levels of insulin and C-peptide concentrations at presentation are highly suggestive of T2DM.

   d Lifestyle modification, including nutrition and exercise advice, is a highly effective intervention in T2DM in adolescents.

   e Metformin is the preferred first-line drug in children with T2DM.

60 Which of the following is not associated with short stature?

   a Silver–Russell's syndrome

   b Turner's syndrome

   c Cystic fibrosis

   d Beckwith–Wiedemann's syndrome

   e Noonan's syndrome

Bibliography

Ali K, Harnden A, Edge JA. Type 1 diabetes in children. *BMJ*. 2011 Feb 16; **342**: d294.

Brook CGD. Growth hormone: panacea or punishment for short stature? *BMJ*. 1997 Sep 20; **315**(7110): 692–3.

Campbell AGM. Infections. In: Campbell AGM, McIntosh N, editors. *Forfar and Arneil's Textbook of Pediatrics*. 5th ed. New York, NY: Churchill Livingstone; 1998. pp. 1273–543.

Copeland KC, Silverstein J, Moore KR, *et al.* Management of newly diagnosed type 2 Diabetes Mellitus (T2DM) in children and adolescents. *Pediatrics*. 2013 Feb; **131**(2): 364–82. Epub 2013 Jan 28.

Daneman D. Type 1 diabetes. *Lancet*. 2006 Mar 11; **367**(9513): 847–58.

Dattani MT, Preece MA. Physical growth and development. In: Campbell AGM, McIntosh N, editors. *Forfar and Arneil's Textbook of Pediatrics*. 5th ed. New York, NY: Churchill Livingstone; 1998. pp. 349–80.

De Kort H, de Koning EJ, Rabelink TJ, *et al.* Islet transplantation in type 1 diabetes. *BMJ*. 2011 Jan 21; **342**: d217.

Deodati A, Cianfarani S. Impact of growth hormone therapy on adult height of children with idiopathic short stature: systematic review. *BMJ*. 2011 Mar 11; **342**: c7157.

Diabetes Control and Complications Trial/Epidemiology of Diabetes Interventions and Complications Research Group. Retinopathy and nephropathy in patients with type 1 diabetes four years after a trial of intensive insulin therapy. *N Engl J Med*. 2000 Feb 10; **342**(6): 381–9.

Diabetes Control and Complications Trial Research Group. Effect of intensive diabetes treatment on the development and progression of long-term complications in adolescents with insulin-dependent diabetes mellitus: Diabetes Control and Complications Trial. *J Pediatr.* 1994 Aug; **125**(2): 177–88.

Garden A. Gynecological diseases. In: Campbell AGM, McIntosh N, editors. *Forfar and Arneil's Textbook of Pediatrics.* 5th ed. New York, NY: Churchill Livingstone; 1998. pp. 985–95.

Gregory JW. What are the main research findings during the last 5 years that have changed my clinical practice in diabetes medicine? *Arch Dis Child.* 2012 May; **97**(5): 436–9. Epub 2011 Nov 18.

Kaufman FR. Intensive management of type 1 diabetes in young children. *Lancet.* 2005 Feb 26–Mar 4; **365**(9461): 737–8.

Kelnar CJH. Endocrine gland disorders and disorders of growth and puberty. In: Campbell AGM, McIntosh N, editors. *Forfar and Arneil's Textbook of Pediatrics.* 5th ed. New York, NY: Churchill Livingstone; 1998. pp. 996–1098.

Lee MM. Clinical practice: idiopathic short stature. *N Engl J Med.* 2006 Jun 15; **354**(24): 2576–82.

Neonatal jaundice

Your next scheduled morning home visit is for 4-day-old baby Eesa. Eesa's mum, originally from Lebanon, opted for a home birth, which went remarkably well. Eesa is being breastfed. He was born at 37 weeks' gestation and there were no immediate complications. Over the last 2 days mum has been struggling to feed Eesa, as she finds that he is not sucking as well as her previous child and he seems to be sleeping all the time. He has had no fever and has had a few wet nappies over the last 24 hours. His urine and stool are of normal colour. He has no rashes and has not been vomiting. As you handle Eesa you notice that he has slightly reduced body tone and has yellowing of the sclera. He is dark skinned, so you ask mum's permission to examine him under natural light. As you carry him close to the window you notice yellowing of his skin on blanching. You organise an immediate split bilirubin blood test. A few hours later the laboratory rings you with the following results.

- *conjugated bilirubin level 4 µmol/L (normal range <8 µmol/L)*
- *unconjugated bilirubin level 420 µmol/L.*

Which of the following is/are *true*?

a   Mum should be reassured that Eesa is suffering from jaundice typical of breastfed babies and he should be kept near the window, in natural daylight, which should resolve the problem.

b   Eesa should be referred immediately to the neonatal team for considera-
    tion of treatment.

c   The extent of hyperbilirubinaemia can be confidently estimated from the
    degree of caudal progression of visible jaundice from the face downwards.

d   Mum should be encouraged to stop breastfeeding and switch to formula
    milk.

e   Gestational age of less than 38 weeks is associated with a greater risk of
    significant hyperbilirubinaemia.

Answer: b and e

The desire to avoid acute bilirubin encephalopathy underpins the management of neonatal jaundice. Bilirubin is the natural breakdown product of
haem. A mild rise in unconjugated bilirubin levels is a normal physiological
phenomenon resulting from increased red cell breakdown and immature
liver function in the neonate. Jaundice becomes clinically apparent, usually
on the second or third day of life, if the bilirubin level rises above 85 µmol/L.
The child usually remains well and the jaundice settles over the course of
7–10 days. However, for various reasons, the bilirubin can exceed normal
physiological levels and become potentially dangerous to the newborn
infant. A build-up of bilirubin in the bloodstream results in the bilirubin
spilling over into brain tissue and causing toxic damage to the basal ganglia
and other brainstem nuclei. Acute bilirubin encephalopathy, also referred to
as kernicterus (although some prefer to use this term to describe the long-
term, chronic neurological sequelae of bilirubin toxicity), remains a rare but
devastating condition. In the early phase, presentation may be non-specific
with lethargy, hypotonia and poor feeding. As the condition progresses
the infant becomes irritable, hypertonic with retrocollis and opisthotonos
(backward arching of neck and back, respectively), develops a shrill high-
pitched cry and may develop a fever. In the latter stages seizures, coma and,
ultimately, death may occur. It is important to recognise and intervene at the
early stages to prevent further progression of the clinical condition. Infants
who survive excessive hyperbilirubinaemia may develop permanent brain

damage in the form of athetoid cerebral palsy, along with other physical and mental handicaps.

Until recently, no guidelines on how to manage elevated unconjugated bilirubin levels in the infant existed. This resulted in a variety of practices being prevalent in different parts of the UK. In 2010, the National Institute for Health and Care Excellence (NICE) issued guidance on how to identify, monitor and manage infants with jaundice. It is important for GPs, health visitors and paediatricians to be familiar with this guideline to help early identification and intervention and allow a similar standard of care through-out the UK.

First, it is important to be on the lookout for jaundice, particularly in high-risk infants. Infants born before 38 weeks of completed gestation, those with a sibling with a history of jaundice and exclusively breastfed infants are all at a greater risk of developing jaundice. If suspected, the infant should be examined naked in bright natural light. Blanching of the skin tends to reveal the true underlying colour. Similarly, a yellow tinge to the sclera may be noted. Accurate estimations of bilirubin levels on visual inspection are not possible. If jaundice is suspected on visual inspection, a formal measurement of bilirubin levels should follow. This can be done by measuring serum levels or via a transcutaneous measurement obtained using a transcutaneous bilirubinometer. This allows bilirubin levels to be measured by placing the device over the sternum or forehead. It has the obvious advantage of being non-invasive. Its use, however, is limited by its availability and by the fact that it should be used only in infants over the age of 35 gestational weeks who are more than 24 hours old. NICE guidelines recommend that if a transcutaneous bilirubin reading is greater than 250 µmol/L then a serum bilirubin level be obtained to confirm the level. Serum readings are also preferred in infants in whom bilirubin levels are being tracked by repeated measurements (due to initially high levels) and in those receiving phototherapy.

Once a bilirubin level is obtained, it is plotted on a graph. The laboratory in the case outlined here is not being difficult by not giving a normal range for the unconjugated bilirubin level. The result needs to be interpreted in conjunction with the child's gestational and actual age. The guidance from

NICE provides a range of charts for infants of gestational ages ranging from 23 to 38 weeks and above. The correct chart for the child should be printed off and placed in the child's notes. The x-axis covers the first 14 days of the child's life. The bilirubin level is plotted on the y-axis. A blue and a red line indicate the two available treatment thresholds. If the bilirubin level falls above the blue line, phototherapy should be considered. If the bilirubin level falls above the red line, then exchange transfusion is the recommended treatment. These treatments are carried out in hospital, hence necessitating a paediatric or neonatal referral, as is locally appropriate. Otherwise, if the child is well and the bilirubin levels are below the treatment threshold, the child can be safely followed up in the community. If the child develops signs and symptoms of acute bilirubin encephalopathy, it should be referred immediately for consideration of exchange transfusion. Raised bilirubin levels requiring treatment are likely to result in further investigations to rule out pathological causes of jaundice.

Eesa may well be suffering from the early effects of acute bilirubin encephalopathy. An immediate blood test is certainly indicated; however, if there are serious concerns regarding the well-being of the child, the child should be referred to hospital as an emergency where the blood test can be carried out while being closely monitored by specialist teams. At such an early age it is difficult to differentiate between various causes of drowsiness, hypotonia and reduced feeding. The unconjugated bilirubin level in this case is high enough to be the culprit necessitating immediate treatment. Exposing the child to natural daylight is appropriate in milder cases of hyperbilirubinaemia. Breastfeeding should be continued, even in children receiving phototherapy.

Infants who present with jaundice in the first 24 hours of their life or beyond 14 days usually require further investigations. Jaundice in the first 24 hours is likely to represent haemolytic disease of the newborn, congenital or postnatal infection, excessive red cell breakdown (e.g. due to a cephalhae-matoma) or rare deficiencies of enzymes involved in bilirubin metabolism. Jaundice persisting beyond 14 days may still be physiological breast milk jaundice but may represent persistent infection, serious liver disease, galac-tosaemia (inability to metabolise galactose) or thyroid problems. When bilirubin levels are measured, the laboratory will normally report back with conjugated and unconjugated levels. A rise in conjugated levels, although not dangerous, is almost always indicative of disease.

Examination practice: neonatal jaundice

Options for questions 61–63:

a glucose-6-phosphate-dehydrogenase deficiency

b galactosaemia

c Gilbert's syndrome

d Alagille's syndrome

e biliary atresia

f Budd–Chiari's syndrome

g choledochal cyst

h Crigler–Najjar's syndrome

i cystic fibrosis

j breast milk jaundice.

The children in questions 61–63 present with conjugated hyperbilirubi-naemia. Based on the additional features described, choose the most likely diagnosis from the list of options provided. Each option may be used once, more than once or not at all.

61 A week-old child with a broad forehead, recessed eyes and a small, pointed chin. An echocardiogram reveals pulmonary stenosis.

62 An ultrasound scan performed on a 3-month-old child reveals an enlarged liver with a very small gall bladder. The ultrasonographer reports a positive 'triangular cord sign' due to a hyperechogenic liver hilum.

63 Mum says that she gets a salty taste in her mouth when she kisses her child and wonders whether it is related to his jaundice.

64 Which of the following statements regarding Apgar score is/are *false*?

a Apgar score measurements are the most widely used method to diagnose asphyxia at birth.

b Four different variables are assessed, usually at 1 and 5 minutes after birth, to give a score of 0–10.

c Almost all children who develop cerebral palsy later in life have Apgar scores of below 5 at 5 minutes.

d Gestational age of the child may depress the Apgar score in the absence of asphyxia.

e An Apgar score of 3 and below is related to an increased risk of death in a full-term infant.

65 The use of which drug in children has been linked with the development of Reye's syndrome?

a Paracetamol

b Codeine

c Isoniazid

d Fluoxetine

e Aspirin

Bibliography

Atkinson M, Budge H. Review of the NICE guidance on neonatal jaundice. *Arch Dis Child Educ Pract Ed*. 2011 Aug; **96**(4): 136–40.

Bisset WM. Disorders of the alimentary tract and liver. In: Campbell AGM, McIntosh N, editors. *Forfar and Arneil's Textbook of Pediatrics*. 5th ed. New York, NY: Churchill Livingstone; 1998. pp. 423–88.

Gilmour SM. Prolonged neonatal jaundice: when to worry and what to do. *Paediatr Child Health*. 2004 Dec; **9**(10): 700–4.

Hartley JL, Davenport M, Kelly DA. Biliary atresia. *Lancet*. 2009 Nov 14; **374**(9702): 1704–13.

McIntosh N. The newborn. In: Campbell AGM, McIntosh N, editors. *Forfar and Arneil's Textbook of Pediatrics*. 5th ed. New York, NY: Churchill Livingstone; 1998. pp. 93–325.

McKenzie S, Silverman M. Respiratory disorders. In: Campbell AGM, McIntosh N, editors. *Forfar and Arneil's Textbook of Pediatrics*. 5th ed. New York, NY: Churchill Livingstone; 1998. pp. 489–583.

Medicines and Healthcare products Regulatory Agency (MHRA). *Press Release: new advice on oral salicylate gels in under 16s*. London: MHRA; 23 April 2009. Available at: www.mhra.gov.uk/NewsCentre/Pressreleases/CON044014 (accessed 24 September 2013).

Nelson KB, Ellenberg JH. Apgar scores as predictors of chronic neurologic disability. *Pediatrics*. 1981 Jul; **68**(1): 36–44.

National Institute for Health and Care Excellence. *Neonatal Jaundice: NICE clinical guideline 98*. London: NICE; 2010. www.nice.org.uk/cg98

Rennie JM, Sehgal A, De A, *et al.* Range of UK practice regarding thresholds for phototherapy and exchange transfusion in neonatal hyperbilirubinaemia. *Arch Dis Child Fetal Neonatal Ed.* 2009 Sep; **94**(5): F323–7. Epub 2008 Nov 10.

Schrör K. Aspirin and Reye syndrome: a review of the evidence. *Paediatr Drugs.* 2007; **9**(3): 195–204.

Recurrent abdominal pain

Eight-year-old Emily is back in your clinic again with her third episode of abdominal pain in 3 months. Since the previous night she has been getting griping central abdominal pains associated with flatulence and repeated visits to the toilet. Defecation seems to ease the pain for a short period but then the pain returns again. She describes her stool as a little loose but denies diarrhoea. She has no fever and the pain is similar in nature to the episode she had the previous month. She (and the rest of the family) has been up all night with it. You note that she went through a similar phase 6 months ago when she would frequently attend the surgery with similar symptoms. All investigations (full blood count, renal and liver function, erythrocyte sedimentation rate, coeliac screen and urine and stool microscopy) had been normal and Emily had continued to gain weight at a satisfactory rate. Mum would like Emily to be referred for a 'scan', as 'something must be wrong'. These recurring episodes are affecting Emily's attendance at school and causing a lot of stress at home too.

Which of the following statement(s) is/are *true*?

a   An ultrasound scan of the abdomen is unlikely to yield a positive result in this case.

b   The underlying cause of Emily's pain is likely to be a complicated interplay between biological, social and psychological factors.

c Original studies by John Apley into recurrent abdominal pain (RAP) of childhood estimated an underlying organic cause in 30% of children.

d Emily should be prescribed a trial of pizotifen, as there is evidence of its benefit in such cases of abdominal pain.

e An increasing body of evidence supports the withdrawal of lactose from the diet to help with Emily's recurring abdominal pain.

Answer: a and b

John Apley first described RAP in 1958 (Apley and Naish, 1958). In this landmark study, which looked at 1000 children at primary and secondary schools in Bristol (hence, making it very relevant to general practice), recurrent abdominal pain was defined as at least three bouts of abdominal pain, severe enough to cause functional impairment in the child, over a period of 3 months. The purpose of the study was to identify the type of children who get abdominal pain. Although conducted over 50 years ago, the study remains an interesting and remarkably valid review of the problem. The study showed a slightly increased prevalence among girls (12.3% vs. 9.5%) with a peak occurring (in girls) between the ages of 8 and 10 years. Apley found the children who suffered from RAP were more likely to be 'highly-strung, fussy, excitable, anxious, timid and apprehensive'. He also observed that they were more likely to have undue fears, suffer from nocturnal enuresis, sleep disorders and have appetite difficulties. Approaching the matter holistically, Apley was keen to determine a profile of the family of the child suffering from RAP. He found that parents and siblings of children who suffer from RAP were more likely to have suffered from RAP themselves. In the majority of these cases the family member would be the mother. Other common family complaints were migraines, history of peptic ulcer and 'nervous breakdowns'. The majority of the children complained of pain in and around the umbilicus. Other reported associated disturbances were pallor, vomiting, fever, headache and subsequent sleepiness or lethargy.

Fifty years on and RAP remains a challenging condition to manage.

Subsequent studies estimate a higher prevalence, ranging from 11% to 45%. Apley dealt with all cases of abdominal pain as a single entity. Later studies have attempted to sub-classify RAP in children based on the clinical symptoms and possible underlying causes. This allows for management strategies based on the likely underlying cause of the pain. The five sub-classifications are illustrated in Figure 4. These sub-classifications (based on the Rome II criteria) require symptoms to be present for at least 12 weeks in the preceding 12 months (at least three episodes in the last 12 months in the case of abdominal migraine) for the diagnosis to be made.

The first step in dealing with RAP is to rule out an underlying organic problem. Primary care physicians now have access to a greater number of investigations than Apley did 50 years ago. This allows a more complete assessment of the problem but also, unfortunately, may identify minor, insignificant problems, which can result in unnecessary anxiety and treatment for the child. Organic disease is thought to account for 5%–10% of cases of RAP in the community. However, other studies, particularly those carried out on children referred to secondary care, have found organic pathology to be much more common. El-Matary, *et al.* (2004) looked at 103 children with RAP and found that organic disease accounted for a third of cases. Apart from a detailed questionnaire and full physical examination, all children were screened for coeliac disease and *Helicobacter pylori* infection and had a full blood count, inflammatory markers, serum amylase, liver function test, stool and urine analysis and an abdominal ultrasound performed. A history suggestive of gastro-oesophageal reflux disease resulted in endoscopy and oesophageal pH monitoring. A history of abdominal pain at night and abdominal tenderness on clinical examination was more likely to be associated with an organic underlying cause. Like Apley, they found abdominal pain that was centred on the umbilicus was less likely to be due to an organic cause. Some of the more organic causes identified in various studies include *H. pylori* infection, a slow transit gut, urinary tract infections and disorders, constipation, gastro-oesophageal reflux disease, coeliac disease and food intolerance. Stool, urine and serum analysis (with the addition of serum glucose measurement to the list given earlier) is not an unreasonable set of initial investigations. Further investigations and referral to secondary care

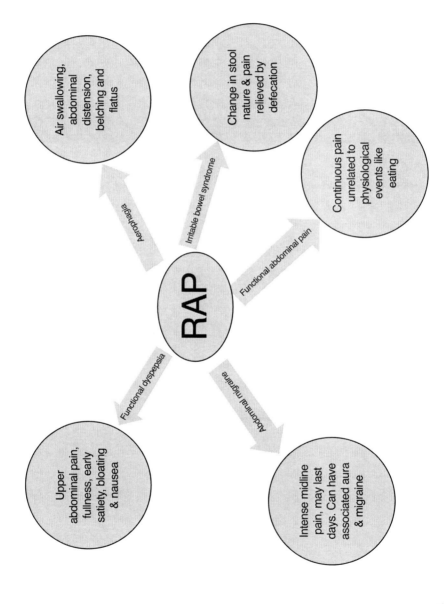

RAP

Aerophagia → Air swallowing, abdominal distension, belching and flatus

Irritable bowel syndrome → Change in stool nature & pain relieved by defecation

Functional abdominal pain → Continuous pain unrelated to physiological events like eating

Functional dyspepsia → Upper abdominal pain, fullness, early satiety, bloating & nausea

Abdominal migraine → Intense midline pain, may last days. Can have associated aura & migraine

FIGURE 4

will generally depend upon the results, course of abdominal pain after initial reassurance and extent of parental concern.

The mainstay of management in RAP is reassurance. Many parents and children are reassured by an explanation and a normal set of initial investigations. Therapeutic options may be classified as pharmacological, psychosocial and dietary. The success of pharmacological therapy may be determined by the underlying cause of the pain. Simple analgesics may be used during flare-ups. Parents should be advised not to give analgesia 'prophylactically', as RAP is a fluctuating condition and natural pain-free days should not be attributed to the analgesic drugs. The serotonin antagonist pizotifen has been shown to be effective in the prophylaxis of abdominal migraine. Symon and Russell (1995) looked at 16 children between the ages of 5 and 13 and found that children receiving pizotifen had fewer days of abdominal pain. Two children reported side effects: drowsiness and weight gain. Another trial (See, *et al.*, 2001) reported a subjective benefit in children with RAP and dyspepsia when treated with H_2-receptor antagonist famotidine compared with placebo. Only 25 children were included in this study. Kline, *et al.* (2001) reported a benefit in 75% of the 42 children recruited in their study, when treated with peppermint oil for irritable bowel syndrome (IBS). These are the only three trials included in the most recent Cochrane review of pharmacological interventions for RAP. Hence, options for pharmacological interventions with good evidence base are limited in RAP. A more helpful approach would be to consider RAP in the context of a biopsychosocial model of disease. Although there may be underlying biological mechanisms responsible for the symptoms (e.g. visceral hyperalgesia, gut dysmotility, autonomic nervous system instability), it is more likely that they are a manifestation of a complex interplay between underlying biology, the child's psychological make-up and social interactions within the family and school environment. As a result, psychological interventions such as cognitive behavioural therapy and family therapy have been tried with some success in RAP. Access to such interventions is generally limited, making it difficult for them to be routinely used. Despite the lack of good-quality evidence in favour of suggesting diet modification, it remains a commonly used strategy in RAP. Children participating in Apley's original study were specifically asked about their milk drinking habits, as it was felt that excessive consumption might be linked with RAP. Apley found that children who suffered from RAP tended to drink less milk than controls. Subsequent studies (Lebenthal, *et al.*, 1981; Dearlove, *et al.*, 1983) have looked at lactose avoidance as a possible management strategy but have failed to show a benefit. Based on this, a prolonged trial of lactose-free diet cannot be advised, but a short trial may be considered along with other management techniques. An increase in fibre intake may also be suggested, despite unreliable and inconclusive data from clinical studies. Gawrońska, *et al.* (2007) looked at dietary supplementation with *Lactobacillus* sp. in 104 children. Children were classified according to Rome II criteria as having IBS, functional dyspepsia or functional abdominal pain. Children with IBS receiving *Lactobacillus* sp. were more likely to have fewer episodes of pain than those receiving placebo (it did not, however, reduce severity of pain). No differences were found in the functional dyspepsia or functional abdominal pain groups. Success with a single dietary component is unlikely and management should involve getting the child to keep a food and pain diary. Suggestions of additions or avoidance of certain foods can then be based on the information derived from such charts.

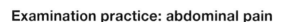

Examination practice: abdominal pain

Options for questions 66–68:

a intussusception

b acute appendicitis

c pyloric stenosis

d haematocolpos

e testicular torsion

f strangulated inguinal hernia

g idiopathic scrotal oedema

h Wilkie's syndrome

i infantile colic.

Questions 66–68 refer to children presenting with abdominal pain. Choose the most appropriate answer from the list provided. Each option may be used once, more than once or not at all.

66 A 15-year-old girl, with normal development of secondary sexual characteristics, presents with amenorrhoea, cyclical abdominal pain and the presence of an abdominal mass.

67 A 6-month-old boy presents with intense crying, drawing up of knees, sporadic vomiting and redcurrant jelly stools. Mum tells you she started weaning him 3 days ago.

68 Hypochloraemic alkalosis is discovered in a 4-week-old girl presenting with worsening vomiting.

69 Which of the following statements regarding male infant circumcision are *true*?

   a Male circumcision is associated with a protective effect against the acquisition of HIV in heterosexual males in areas of high HIV prevalence.

   b There is strong evidence that male circumcision is associated with a reduced risk of developing gonorrhoea and chlamydia.

   c Circumcision appears to be protective against the development of a urinary tract infection in boys under the age of 2.

   d Male circumcision is associated with a lower risk of invasive penile cancer but a slightly increased risk of cervical cancer in the female partner.

e Male infant circumcision is associated with reduced sexual satisfaction and sexual function compared with non-circumcised men.

70 Which of the following tumours is associated with aniridia?

a Neuroblastoma

b Wilms's tumour

c Non-Hodgkin's lymphoma

d Rhabdomyosarcoma

e Ewing's sarcoma

Bibliography

American Academy of Pediatrics Task Force on Circumcision. Male circumcision. *Pediatrics*. 2012 Sep; **130**(3): e756–85. Epub 2012 Aug 27.

Apley J, Naish N. Recurrent abdominal pains: a field survey of 1000 school children. *Arch Dis Child*. 1958 Apr; **33**(168): 165–70.

Ceccuti A. Case report: haematocolpos with imperforate hymen. *Can Med Assoc J*. 1964; **90**(25): 1420–1.

Davidoff AM. Wilms tumor. *Adv Pediatr*. 2012; **59**(1): 247–67.

Dearlove J, Dearlove B, Pearl K, *et al.* Dietary lactose and the child with abdominal pain. *Br Med J* (*Clin Res Ed*). 1983 Jun 18; **286**(6382): 1936.

El-Matary W, Spray C, Sandhu B. Irritable bowel syndrome: the commonest cause of recurrent abdominal pain in children. *Eur J Pediatr*. 2004 Oct; **163**(10): 584–8.

Gawrońska A, Dziechciarz P, Horvath A, *et al.* A randomized double-blind placebo-controlled trial of *Lactobacillus GG* for abdominal pain disorders in children. *Aliment Pharmacol Ther*. 2007 Jan 15; **25**(2): 177–84.

Huertas-Ceballos A, Logan S, Bennett C, *et al.* Dietary interventions for recurrent abdominal pain (RAP) and irritable bowel syndrome (IBS) in childhood. *Cochrane Database Syst Rev*. 2009 Jan 21; (1): CD003019.

Huertas-Ceballos A, Logan S, Bennett C, *et al.* Pharmacological interventions for recurrent abdominal pain (RAP) and irritable bowel syndrome (IBS) in childhood. *Cochrane Database Syst Rev*. 2008 Jan 23; (1): CD003017.

Huertas-Ceballos A, Logan S, Bennett C, *et al.* Psychosocial interventions for recurrent abdominal pain (RAP) and irritable bowel syndrome (IBS) in childhood. *Cochrane Database Syst Rev*. 2008 Jan 23; (1): CD003014.

Hulka F, Campbell TJ, Campbell JR, *et al.* Evolution in the recognition of infantile hypertrophic pyloric stenosis. *Pediatrics*. 1997 Aug; **100**(2): E9.

Kline RM, Kline JJ, Di Palma J, *et al.* Enteric-coated, pH-dependent peppermint oil capsules for the treatment of irritable bowel syndrome in children. *J Pediatr*. 2001 Jan; **138**(1): 125–8.

Lebenthal E, Rossi TM, Nord KS, *et al.* Recurrent abdominal pain and lactose absorption in children. *Pediatrics*. 1981 Jun; **67**(6): 828–32.

Liberman M, Daily B. *Paediatrics: what shall I do?* Oxford: Butterworth-Heinemann; 1993.

MacKinlay GA, Watson ACH. Surgical paediatrics. In: Campbell AGM, McIntosh N, editors. *Forfar and Arneil's Textbook of Pediatrics*. 5th ed. New York, NY: Churchill Livingstone; 1998. pp. 1768–801.

Plunkett A, Beattie RM. Recurrent abdominal pain in childhood. *J R Soc Med*. 2005 Mar; **98**(3): 101–6.

Razaq S. *Difficult Cases in Primary Care: women's health*. London: Radcliffe Publishing; 2012.

See MC, Birnbaum AH, Schechter CB, *et al.* Double-blind, placebo-controlled trial of famotidine in children with abdominal pain and dyspepsia: global and quantitative assessment. *Dig Dis Sci*. 2001 May; **46**(5): 985–92.

Symon DN, Russell G. Double blind placebo controlled trial of pizotifen syrup in the treatment of abdominal migraine. *Arch Dis Child*. 1995 Jan; **72**(1): 48–50.

Weydert JA, Ball TM, Davis MF. Systematic review of treatments for recurrent abdominal pain. *Pediatrics*. 2003 Jan; **111**(1): e1–11.

Wheeler R, Malone P. Male circumcision: risk versus benefit. *Arch Dis Child*. 2013 May; **98**(5): 321–2. Epub 2013 Jan 29.

Juvenile idiopathic arthritis

Five-year-old Amal presents with a 1-week history of intermittent limping and knee swelling. Mum tells you that she has been suffering from a cold but this has not bothered her. Amal has missed the last week from school, as she has been finding it difficult to 'get going' in the morning. Mum initially thought this might be due to problems at school but a chat with Amal's teacher revealed no problems. Mum has been more concerned lately, as the limping seems to persist all day and mum has noticed Amal's right knee to be swollen at times. Amal herself is unable to localise the pain and just says that her right leg hurts. On examination you fail to elicit any swelling in the knees or any other joints and note a normal range of movements in clinic. Amal is afebrile and well, has no rashes and there is no preceding history of trauma. You organise a precautionary blood test for a full blood count (FBC), C-reactive protein (CRP) and erythrocyte sedimentation rate (ESR), which are reported as normal the following day. You advise mum that this is probably a reactive arthritis secondary to a viral infection and should settle over the next few weeks. Six weeks later mum returns with Amal who now is finding it difficult to walk and has appreciable swelling of both knees and her right ankle. She remains afebrile and systemically well.

Which of the following statements represents the best management plan for Amal?

a   Amal should be prescribed a non-steroidal anti-inflammatory drug and advised complete bed rest for 2 weeks.

b   She should be prescribed 1 mg/kg/day of prednisolone and be reviewed again in 5 days.

c   A repeat FBC, ESR and CRP should be organised and Amal reviewed again when results are available.

d   One should continue to 'watch and wait', as the course is not atypical of reactive arthritis secondary to a viral infection.

e   Amal should be referred to the duty paediatric team for further assessment.

Answer: e

Amal is likely to be suffering from oligoarthritis, a reasonably well-defined category of juvenile idiopathic arthritis (JIA) based on a certain set of clinical features and, therefore, warrants paediatric assessment for further investigations. JIA is a generic term used to describe a number of clinically different arthritides in children of unknown cause. Persistence of symptoms for more than 6 weeks in a child under the age of 16 is required for diagnosis. Figure 5 shows the various categories of JIA with their estimated frequency ranges. These subsets are based on clinical criteria and represent an effort by the International League of Associations for Rheumatology to standardise JIA nomenclature to allow effective collaboration in international research and provide useful prognostic data. The classification system, however, is far from perfect and remains a work in progress.

JIA is the most common chronic rheumatology disease in children. There is a possibility that the true prevalence of the condition is being underestimated, possibly as a result of under-recognition. Missed or late diagnosis can be a cause of considerable short- and long-term disability. It is therefore imperative that the primary care physician is familiar with the various clinical presentations of JIA to facilitate prompt diagnosis, intervention and management. **Oligoarthritis** is the most commonly described subset

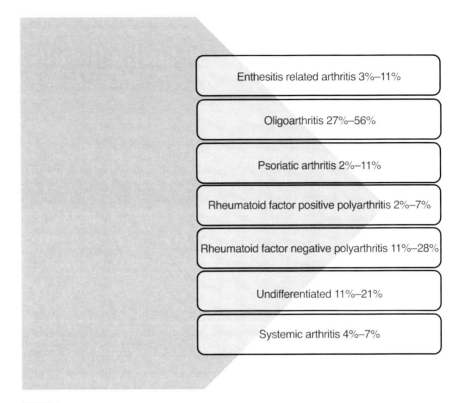

Enthesitis related arthritis 3%–11%

Oligoarthritis 27%–56%

Psoriatic arthritis 2%–11%

Rheumatoid factor positive polyarthritis 2%–7%

Rheumatoid factor negative polyarthritis 11%–28%

Undifferentiated 11%–21%

Systemic arthritis 4%–7%

FIGURE 5

of JIA. It accounts for approximately half of all the cases of JIA. It is more common in girls and is defined as an arthritis affecting four or fewer joints during the initial 6 months of the disease course. The child would still be considered to have oligoarthritis if, after the first 6 months, further joints were to be involved. It primarily affects the lower limbs with the knee joint most commonly affected. Initial investigation may reveal a markedly raised ESR. A large proportion of patients will have considerably high titres of antinuclear antibodies, which is a risk factor for developing iridocyclitis, one of the complications of oligoarthritis. This is a chronic form of anterior uveitis in which there is inflammation of the iris and ciliary body, which can cause significant visual disability. All children with oligoarthritis should be routinely and regularly screened for iridocyclitis with a slit lamp examination. **Systemic arthritis** is the paediatric form of adult-onset Still's disease. Clinical features include quotidian fever (intermittent daily spikes of temperature) of at least 2 weeks' duration, salmon-coloured erythematosus rash that comes and goes (typically with the fever spikes or after a hot bath), hepatomegaly or splenomegaly (or both), serositis and lymphadenopathy. Diagnosing systemic arthritis can be challenging, as the arthritis (usually polyarticular and symmetrical) may not appear for weeks after the onset of systemic symptoms. It can be a cause of significant morbidity and mortality, particularly if a rare complication of the condition, macrophage activation syndrome, develops. Activated macrophages consume haematopoietic cells in the bone marrow causing organ failure, coagulopathy, encephalopathy, seizures and possible death. **Rheumatoid factor (RF)-positive polyarthritis** is the same as adult RF-positive disease and is arthritis involving five or more joints in the first 6 months of disease. As in adults the small joints of the hands and feet are symmetrically involved and rheumatoid nodules may be seen. Diagnosis requires a positive IgM RF on two separate occasions at least 3 months apart. **RF-negative polyarthritis** is a less well-defined clinical subset in which five or more joints are affected in the first 6 months with a negative IgM RF result. In some cases this subset may mimic oligoarthritis or even RF-positive polyarthritis in its clinical course. **Enthesitis-related arthritis** (as the name suggests) describes a clinical subset of JIA in which joint and entheses (sites of tendon or ligament attachment to bone) inflammation is associated with each other. This subset of JIA belongs to the spondyloarthropathy group of disorders – of which, ankylosing spondylitis is the best-studied example. Arthritis presenting with a typical psoriatic rash describes the sixth subset of JIA, **psoriatic arthritis**. A diagnosis of psoriatic arthritis may also be made in the absence of the rash if there is a family history of psoriasis in a first-degree relative, nail pitting or onycholysis or dactylitis (two of the three needed along with arthritis). Currently, all children who do not fulfil the criteria for any of the described subsets or fulfil the criteria for more than one of the subsets are classified as having **undifferentiated arthritis**.

Despite recent advances in the understanding of the aetiopathogenesis of JIA, it remains a poorly understood condition. Infective triggers are attractive causative culprits but there is little evidence to substantiate this claim.

It is likely that a host of environmental and genetic factors play contributory roles in the development of JIA. The growing skeleton of the child is a double-edged sword in the management of JIA. Whereas deformities in adults with rheumatoid arthritis are generally permanent, a child may recover from any damage, because of post-treatment restoration in the growing skeleton. On the flip side, however, if the active inflammation arrests growth in the growth plate then skeletal abnormalities such as leg length discrepancy and micrognathia may develop. Therapeutic approaches are determined by the extent and severity of disease but are likely to include pharmacotherapy, physiotherapy, occupational therapy, psychological support and surgery. Rest is important, and in some cases unavoidable, but parents should be discouraged from being overprotective of their children. Participation in normal activities is essential for the child to develop self-confidence and to prevent assumption of the 'sick role'. Excessive angiogenesis and hyperplasia of the synovium is seen in active disease and newer therapies have evolved, specifically targeting the molecular components driving these inflammatory processes. The aim of treatment is to eliminate inflammation in the joint, preserving normal function, so that long-term deformity and disability may be prevented. Drug options include non-steroidal anti-inflammatory drugs (e.g. naproxen, indomethacin, ibuprofen), intra-articular or systemic steroids, disease-modifying anti-rheumatic drugs (e.g. methotrexate) and biological agents. The aim of physiotherapy is to keep the joints mobile and maintain good strength. Children should be encouraged to move all joints. Parents may wish to sit the child in a hot bath to ease the stiffness and allow easy movements of the joints. Children should be encouraged to exercise, sticking to disciplines that result in minimal stress on the joints (e.g. cycling and swimming). Competitive contact sports such as football and rugby should be avoided, particularly in active disease. Occupational therapy is aimed at keeping the child as independent as possible, helping with daily activities. For the most severely impaired by the arthritis, surgical intervention is an option but it is usually delayed until after growth has halted.

Examination practice: limb pain

Options for questions 71–73:

a septic arthritis

b transient synovitis of the hip

c Perthes's disease

d developmental dysplasia of the hip

e slipped upper femoral epiphysis

f Lyme arthritis

g non-accidental injury

h malignancy

i Köhler's disease.

Questions 71–73 refer to children presenting with limb pain. Choose the most appropriate answer from the options provided. Each answer may be used once, more than once or not at all.

71 A 7-year-old boy presents with a 1-year history of a limp and leg pain on activity. X-ray of the hip reveals widening of the joint space and flattening of a sclerosed femoral head, suggesting early avascular necrosis of the femoral head.

72 A 3-year-old girl presents with fever and inability to bear weight over the preceding 48 hours. Blood tests reveal a raised ESR and CRP.

73 An 11-year-old boy presents with an acute onset of limb pain after a twisting injury in the playground. On examination he finds it difficult to move the affected leg and holds it in an externally rotated position. He weighs 70 kg.

74 Which of the following statements regarding Duchenne's muscular dystrophy (DMD) are *true*?

a DMD is inherited in an autosomal dominant fashion.

b DMD occurs exclusively in males.

c Diagnosis is clinical, with a positive Gower's sign confirming the diagnosis.

d Prognosis is good, with most males remaining independent till the fourth decade of their life.

e Creatine phosphokinase (CPK) estimation is rarely useful, as it is often normal in early stages of muscle destruction.

75 Which one of the following is *not* a major manifestation of the Jones criteria for the diagnosis of rheumatic fever?

a Carditis

b Polyarthritis

c Sydenham's chorea

d Erythema multiforme

e Subcutaneous nodules

Bibliography

Barr DGD, Crofton PM, Goel KM. Disorders of bone, joints and connective tissue. In: Campbell AGM, McIntosh N, editors. *Forfar and Arneil's Textbook of Pediatrics*. 5th ed. New York, NY: Churchill Livingstone; 1998. pp. 1544–615.

Brown JK, Minns RA. Disorders of the central nervous system. Surgical paediatrics. In: Campbell AGM, McIntosh N, editors. *Forfar and Arneil's Textbook of Pediatrics*. 5th ed. New York, NY: Churchill Livingstone; 1998. pp. 641–846.

Caird MS, Flynn JM, Leung YL, *et al.* Factors distinguishing septic arthritis from transient synovitis of the hip in children: a prospective study. *J Bone Joint Surg Am*. 2006 Jun; **88**(6): 1251–7.

Ferrier P, Bamatter F, David Klein D. Muscular dystrophy (Duchenne) in a girl with Turner's syndrome. *J Med Genet*. 1965 March; **2**(1): 38–46.

Kahn P. Juvenile idiopathic arthritis: an update on pharmacotherapy. *Bull NYU Hosp Jt Dis*. 2011; **69**(3): 264–76.

Ravelli A, Martini A. Juvenile idiopathic arthritis. *Lancet*. 2007 Mar 3; **369**(9563): 767–78.

Smith E, Anderson M, Foster H. The child with a limp: a symptom and not a diagnosis. *Arch Dis Child Educ Pract Ed*. 2012 Oct; **97**(5): 185–93. Epub 2012 Jul 21.

Answers

1   f

Angelman's syndrome is a rare condition associated with epilepsy, severe learning disabilities and speech difficulties. The child's stiff, puppet-like gait and vertical ataxia resulted in this being known as 'happy puppet syndrome'. Facial features include prognathism (bulging out of the mandible), tongue protrusion and a hooked nose. The child is noted to have a happy demeanour with sudden out-bursts of laughter, resulting in a delay in diagnosis until such behaviours become apparent. West's syndrome is part of a distinctive group of epilepsy syndromes termed 'malignant epileptic syndromes'. They are remarkably resistant to anti-epileptic treatment and have a high seizure frequency. Cognition may be impaired and a progressive dementia may develop.

2   e

Benign rolandic epilepsy is among the commonest types of epilepsy in children. The child usually presents with the described abnormal neurology upon wak-ing. The speech can be affected if seizure activity affects the throat. Drooling may be present. Seizure activity may progress to cause tonic–clonic seizures of the face and limbs on the same side. Occasionally the seizure may become generalised resulting in loss of consciousness and postictal confusion. An EEG may show centrotemporal spikes, a feature that is usually associated with a more favourable prognosis. Overall, in most children seizures will settle by the time the child reaches puberty. If seizures are frequent, anti-epileptic medication may be prescribed. Carbamazepine, lamotrigine and sodium valproate are effective options available.

3   b

Breath-holding attacks are a benign, non-harmful 'funny turn' usually triggered by emotional upset. Temper tantrums, pain from knocking oneself or excessive crying may trigger a short period of the child not breathing. This may result in the child looking pale and occasionally cyanosed. If normal breathing does not resume the child may lose consciousness for a few seconds. Very rarely, it may result in a seizure. Reassurance of the parents is all that is needed, as most children will grow out of breath-holding attacks before joining school. Pavor nocturnus, more commonly known as night terrors, is a sleep disorder that can run in families. The child may wake screaming and frightened, with little or no recall of the cause afterwards.

4   a, c, d and e

Retinoblastoma is the commonest primary eye tumour in children, accounting for approximately 3% of all childhood cancers. Although it is a life-threatening condition, prognosis is excellent, particularly when identified early, with 98% of children surviving the condition in the UK. However, recent campaigns have unfortunately displayed that there is usually a delay in diagnosis of retinoblastoma. This may be due to a lack of awareness of the presenting signs and symptoms of the condition in primary care or a low index of suspicion. Important signs and symptoms include an absence of the red reflex, an intermittent white pupillary reflex (leukocoria), strabismus, change in the colour of the iris, a worsening of vision and unexplained redness and soreness of the eye. A delayed diagnosis increases the risk of extraocular disease and the need for more aggressive treatment. Recent advances in genetics have revealed a genetic form of retinoblastoma linked to mutations in the RB1 gene. Children with this hereditary form of retinoblastoma are at increased risk of developing other forms of cancer later in life. These may occur anywhere in the body. Patients should be advised to avoid smoking and ultraviolet light (because of the risk of malignant melanoma). Extra care should be taken to avoid unnecessary irradiation from X-rays, because of the increased risk in cancer.

5 a

Marfan's syndrome is a connective tissue disorder affecting primarily musculo-skeletal, cardiovascular and ocular systems. Abnormally long limbs and increased flexibility of the joints is seen. Steinberg's sign is positive when the thumb, when enclosed in the fist, protrudes beyond the medial border of the hand. Walker's sign is positive when the little finger and thumb overlap while encircling the con-tralateral wrist. Gower's sign is seen in Duchenne's muscular dystrophy when the child uses his or her hands to climb up his or her legs while getting up. Rovsing's sign is seen in appendicitis where palpation of the left iliac fossa reproduces pain in the right iliac fossa, presumably due to peritoneal irritation. Scarf sign is elicited in the newborn and assesses the tone of the muscles in the upper limbs. Murphy's sign is seen in acute cholecystitis.

6 g

Lead poisoning is rare in the UK. Whereas acute poisoning is an emergency, chronic lead poisoning may present with non-specific symptoms such as con-stipation, irritability, headaches, behavioural problems and abdominal pain. The most common sources of lead exposure in children are deteriorating paint in old houses, contaminated dust and soil and lead pipes in unrefurbished old houses. A history of pica should be sought where lead toxicity is suspected, although blood lead concentrations of 20 µg/dL or greater can be achieved without frank pica. The aim is to bring the blood lead level to below 10 µg/dL. However, recent opinion (Binns, et al., 2007) seems to suggest that harm to the child may occur at lower levels also. For blood lead concentrations below 45 µg/dL, treatment is not always necessary and may just involve regular review and removal of the hazard-ous source of lead. Higher levels necessitate oral or parenteral chelation therapy.

7 b

In the absence of routine surveillance, congenital anorectal abnormalities may be missed. There is a wide range of anorectal anomalies that can occur congenitally. Depending on the type of anomaly, there may be complete anorectal agenesis with or without complicated fistulas between adjacent organs or simply just anal stenosis. Anal stenosis is treated by gradual anal dilation and anoplasty if needed. Prognosis is better if an early diagnosis is made and effective treatment instituted. An abnormality on visual examination may not always be apparent, hence occasionally necessitating a digital rectal exam with the fifth digit.

8   c

Hirschsprung's disease is a congenital neuropathic condition of the intestine characterised by the absence of ganglion cells in the myenteric plexuses of the distal bowel. The aganglionic bowel extends proximally from the rectum for a variable distance, and hence may be classified as short segment (affecting the rectum and/or the sigmoid colon) or long segment (extending beyond the sigmoid). Rarely total colonic aganglionosis may occur affecting the small bowel or even the entire alimentary canal. The exact mechanism of disease is unclear, although some have postulated towards a defect in the migration of ganglion cells from the neural crest between the seventh and eighth week of intrauterine development. Failure or delay in passing meconium (beyond 24 hours), vomiting, abdominal distension and poor feeding are suggestive of Hirschsprung's disease. The presence of diarrhoea may represent Hirschsprung's enterocolitis, a critical complication carrying high rates of mortality. Abdominal radiography and barium enemas are employed in making the diagnosis, although definitive diagnosis is by rectal biopsy. Treatment involves bowel rest, rectal dilation and irrigation, antibiotics and surgery to remove the aganglionic bowel.

9   b, d and e

CF is the commonest genetic inherited disease in the white population and is the commonest cause of severe chronic lung disease in children. It is inherited in an autosomal recessive fashion. Despite its major impact on the lungs, it is a multisystem disease and requires management by multidisciplinary teams in secondary and tertiary centres. Early recognition is vital to prevent a prolonged period of recurrent infections, malabsorption, stunted growth and terminal lung disease. Early, aggressive and multidisciplinary management of CF has lead to a huge improvement in quality of life and longevity. Neonatal screening has helped with this. All neonates have a Guthrie blood test. Neonates with positive results are referred for genetic tests looking for mutations in the cystic fibrosis transmembrane conductance regulator (CFTR) gene. CFTR gene defects (more than 400 have been identified) may lead to defective sodium and chloride transport across epithelial cells, resulting in increased levels of the two ions in surface sweat. This forms the basis of the sweat test. However, some individuals with rarer CF genotypes may have a negative sweat test. These individuals are likely to have milder disease expression also. There is a high incidence of CFTR mutations in men with congenital bilateral absence of the vas deferens, leading to the idea that this condition may be a variant presentation of CF. It is important to note that not all polymorphisms in the CFTR gene cause disease.

10   e

Acute salt loss in CF may lead to the gradual development of abnormally low serum electrolyte levels (hypochloraemia, hypokalaemia and hyponatraemia) and metabolic alkalosis with a failure to thrive. Weight gain resumes with replacement of the lost salts (Kennedy, *et al.*, 1990). Excessive ingestion of milk or calcium carbonate as antacids may lead to hypercalcaemia, alkalosis and renal failure (milk-alkali syndrome). Undiagnosed diabetes, a recognised complication of CF, may result in metabolic acidosis in the form of diabetic ketoacidosis (rather than alkalosis). Pyloric stenosis may cause a similar alkalotic picture and has been discussed elsewhere. It is not a recognised complication of CF. Imerslund–Gräsbeck syndrome is another autosomal recessive disorder, resulting in an inability to absorb vitamin B_{12}.

11   b

12   i

13   h

The three modes of imaging that are the most useful for assessing the urinary tract in a child are ultrasonography, micturating cystourethrogram (MCUG) and renal scintigraphy with DMSA. Ultrasonography is the most non-invasive test and can provide valuable anatomical information regarding the renal tract. It is a useful test that can help identify children who may need further imaging. MCUG is considered the gold standard test for identifying VUR. It involves introduction of a radiopaque, radioactive or echo-contrast medium into the bladder via a catheter. Filling and voiding images are then taken to identify reflux. Not only may it be distressing to the child and parents, it may also introduce infection and cause urethral trauma. Renal scintigraphy involves the intravenous injection of DMSA, which accumulates in renal tissue, to help identify areas of damage. It is performed 4–6 months after the infection so that areas of permanent damage are not confused with areas of acute damage caused by pyelonephritis.

The purpose of imaging is to identify children with renal disease caused by VUR as a result of the UTI. These children can then be treated with prophylactic antibiotics (or surgery in some cases) to prevent the progression of renal disease. Imaging is not indicated in all children after a febrile UTI. The reason for this is that the risk of developing renal scars as a result of a UTI is relatively low. Furthermore, the risk of renal complications as a result of the scarring is even lower. Another compelling reason not to scan every child is that a significant number of children with renal defects (particularly infants) will have been born with the abnormalities. These congenital defects are not amenable to antibiotic prophylaxis. Coupled with the radiation exposure to the child, infection risk associated with certain procedures and the overall cost to the National Health Service of routine scanning, it would be more appropriate to target imaging in children at a greater risk of developing renal complications. The decision to carry out imaging tests under NICE guidelines is based on whether the UTI is uncomplicated (responding to antibiotics within 48 hours), atypical (seriously ill or septic child, non-*E. coli* UTI, not responding to antibiotics within 48 hours, abnormal renal function, poor urine flow or presence of an abdominal mass) or recurrent. If the UTI is uncomplicated, then ultrasonography is indicated only in the infant younger than 6 months old. This should be carried out within 6 weeks. Further imaging may be indicated if the USS is abnormal. Atypical or recurrent UTIs in this age group would warrant an MCUG, DMSA scintigraphy and an urgent USS. In children who are older than 6 months but younger than 3 years, an atypical and recurrent UTI would be an indication for an ultrasound (if the child is unwell, as in Question 13, the USS should be done urgently) and DMSA scintigraphy. An MCUG can be considered in this age group if there is a family history of VUR, the child has abnormal urine flow, dilatation is present on ultrasound or infection is caused by a non-*E. coli* microbe. In children older than 3 years of age, DMSA scintigraphy is recommended only in the context of a recurrent UTI. This is preceded by a routine USS (as in Question 12). An USS should be performed if the infection is atypical, urgently if the child is unwell.

14   a, b and e

Infections, particularly in the winter months, account for the large majority of general practice consultations. Treating infections that need treating (and not treating the ones that do not) while managing patient expectations remains challenging. Previous early use of antibiotics frequently reinforces the idea that 'my sore throat always responds immediately to antibiotics'. However, the case usually is that antibiotics are started at the time of natural resolution of the infection. On the other hand, antibiotics do reduce the incidence of acute otitis media, acute sinusitis and peritonsillar abscess (Del Mar, *et al.*, 2006). With increasing drug resistance patterns, the judicious and appropriate use of antibiotics is as crucial as ever. Traditionally, guidelines have generally opted for longer courses of antibiotics. There is, however, evidence that shorter, high-dose courses are associated with reduced pathogenic resistance. High-dose amoxicillin over 5 days has been shown to reduce the spread of drug-resistant pneumococcus when compared with low-dose amoxicillin over 10 days (Schrag, *et al.*, 2004). A 3-day course is sufficient for an uncomplicated lower UTI. Shorter courses, where possible, are also likely to reduce side effects and encourage better compliance. Osteomyelitis and septic arthritis are treated with longer courses of antibiotics, typically 4 weeks and more. Interestingly, a recent survey of parents' attitudes to childhood fever found that physical examination of the child, information about the underlying cause of the fever and reassurance were the most important things to parents presenting to their GP. Obtaining antibiotics was considered one of the least important priorities during the consultation (de Bont, *et al.*).

15   b

Head lice infection is a common, distressing and often stigmatising infection in the paediatric population. It is caused by the parasite *Pediculus capitis*, with humans being its only known host. The adult female lays eggs on the hair shafts close to the scalp. Nymphs appear from the eggs after 6–10 days and after a series of moults become adult louse over the following 10 days. Untreated, female lice will survive for up to 3 months, laying 5–10 eggs per day. Traditionally, head lice have been treated with neurotoxic pediculicides, which are applied 7 days apart, as they are primarily active against adult louse and nymphs only. The second course allows any untreated eggs to hatch, thus targeting the newly emerging nymphs. Treatment of family members may also be required, because of frequent cross-infection. Contrary to some beliefs, the parasite cannot fly (as it is wingless) and it is unlikely that spread occurs from contaminated garments, as it requires being close to a blood source to survive. Over the years conventional topical pediculicides have become less effective because of emerging patterns of resistance. In some cases efficacy may have dropped to as low as 10%. Dimeticone is a topical non-neurotoxic agent that is thought to work by coating the lice and disrupting their ability to regulate their internal water environment. It should be applied on dry hair and scalp. It should then be left to dry naturally and washed off after 8 hours. The whole process should then be repeated after 7 days. Ivermectin is an oral antiparasitic drug. It works by paralysing the lice by its action on the mediation of neurotransmission by γ-aminobutyric acid (Campbell, *et al.*, 1983). Other possible treatment options include wet combing, plant-based compounds such as tea tree oil and coconut-based compounds, hot air and various electronic devices. However, evidence for their effectiveness is currently scant (Tebruegge, *et al.*, 2010).

16   i

These questions relate to the management of acute and chronic asthma based on the recommendations of the British Thoracic Society and the Scottish Intercollegiate Guidelines Network. The guidelines include a useful step-up diagram to help determine the most suitable management of a child with chronic asthma. The 3-year-old boy in Question 11 is presenting with a moderate exacerbation of acute asthma. Appropriate management in a 3-year-old child would be to give 10 puffs of salbutamol 100 mcg/metered dose via a large-volume spacer or 2.5 mg nebulised salbutamol. Occasionally, usually based on previous experience, parents may insist on a nebuliser because of perceived improved efficacy. A Cochrane database review by Cates, *et al.* (2006) showed that β_2-agonist delivery via a spacer device in children had more benefits over a nebuliser in acute asthma.

Children in whom a spacer device was used had shorter stays in hospital emergency departments and also had lower pulse rates. This is beneficial, as it allows effective advice to be given to parents over the phone when needed. In this case the initial treatment has worked but the child is struggling soon after. As a result the child needs to be referred to hospital immediately for further assessment until adequate control of his breathing can be achieved, as it would be unsafe to monitor in the primary care setting.

17 a

This child represents step one in the management guidelines. He is currently not taking any medication and he appears to wheeze in relation to a viral infection. A lot of the time, treatment is not necessary in these so-called 'happy wheezers'. In such cases the wheeze causes no distress and usually settles on its own accord as the infection runs its course. However, it may be unsettling for the parents. A prompt review usually settles their nerves. If there is suggestion of the wheeze affecting the child's breathing or causing night-time cough then a short-acting β_2-agonist is a reasonable first option. Its use as a reliever for occasional relief should be stressed and if it is being used more than twice a day then a step up to inhaled corticosteroids as preventer therapy should be considered. If inhaled corticosteroids are used and symptom control is achieved then the child should be reviewed, at some stage, to see if stepping down of therapy is appropriate (halving the dose of inhaled corticosteroid is one possibility).

18 i

Paradoxical bronchospasm can be a problem associated with inhaled corticosteroids. A trial of steroid by dry powder inhalation may be considered as an alternative to aerosol inhalers. Another useful way of preventing this is for the β_2-agonist inhalation to precede steroid inhalation to counteract the bronchospasm. The risk of oral candidiasis can be minimised by washing the child's mouth and brushing his or her teeth after steroid inhalation. This child has had two attempts and failed. Montelukast is a leukotriene receptor antagonist and is an effective, well-tolerated alternative where inhaled corticosteroids are not tolerated. This child remains poorly controlled and should be referred to a respiratory paediatrician.

19   a and c

As the name suggests, eczema herpeticum is mostly caused by herpes simplex virus type 1 or 2 and is a potentially fatal complication of atopic eczema in children. Its alternative name, Kaposi's varicelliform eruption, was coined on Kaposi's observations that it looked rather like a chickenpox infection. Other viruses, such as Coxsackie, may also be the underlying cause of the sudden eruption. The child usually presents with fever and systemic unwellness. Glands may be swollen and a blistery rash is seen in areas of eczematous skin. New blisters continue to appear over a period of 7–10 days while old ones crust over. Superinfection with bacteria is not uncommon and can complicate treatment. Eczema herpeticum should be considered a dermatological emergency necessitating referral of the child to specialist paediatric dermatology services. Oral or intravenous antiviral treatment is used depending on response and general condition of the child. Recurrences in children are rare (Liddle, 1990). Preceding treatment of topical steroids is unlikely to be a causative factor. Eczema herpeticum may also be a complication in other conditions in which the skin barrier is faulty (David and Longson, 1985).

20   c

Calculating the expected final height is important when assessing the growth in a child. Recording of height on growth charts in the 'red book' is now standard practice in the UK. Plotting height on the charts helps track normal growth and allows any decelerations in growth to be picked up. Calculation of MPH is useful in estimating the final height a child may achieve. Option b is the formula used for girls. For a boy the target centile range is ±10 cm around the MPH. For a girl the target centile range is ±8.5 cm around the MPH. The figure of 14 represents the average height difference between men and women in the UK. This should be borne in mind when calculating MPH for other populations.

21   c

Pityriasis rosea is a benign, self-limiting rash of unknown aetiology. Not infrequently, it is seen with viral infections, leading many to postulate that the rash is of viral origin. It is commonly seen in children and young adults. Typically, the rash is preceded by a single scaly lesion that may be round or oval in shape. This is known as a 'herald patch' and can easily be confused as a patch of eczema or tinea corporis. A few days later the widespread macular eruption appears, prompting a second (usually more worried) visit to the doctor. The child is usually well and the rash is rarely itchy. Patients should be advised that the rash may be present for 3 months and treatment is neither necessary nor effective. Various treatment modalities including antihistamines, topical steroids and oral antibiotics have been tried but have failed to provide good evidence to support their routine use. Antihistamines, however, may be used if the child complains of itching associated with the rash. Important differential diagnoses include secondary syphilis, guttate psoriasis and cutaneous T-cell lymphoma. Pityriasis versicolor is a rash caused by *Malassezia*, a yeast-like germ.

22 g

Acrodermatitis enteropathica is a rare genetic disease inherited in an autosomal recessive pattern. It is likely that gene mutations result in a defective zinc transporter protein, resulting in reduced uptake from the intestine. This may become apparent when the child is weaned off breast milk, because of low bioavailability of zinc in alternative milk sources and solids. Zinc deficiency may also be acquired in other conditions that cause malabsorption, such as cystic fibrosis. The rash is erythematous and crusted and may be well demarcated from normal skin. The rash can affect the eyes, mouth and nose, tips of fingers, knees and elbows. Hair loss may occur and wound healing can be impaired. Superimposed bacterial and candidal infection may also occur. The genetic form requires lifelong zinc replacement, which results in rapid improvement in the child. Papular acrodermatitis of childhood is a papular eruption affecting the extremities, associated with anicteric hepatitis (raised alanine aminotransferase, normal bilirubin levels). It is thought to be of viral aetiology, with hepatitis B virus particularly implicated.

23 b

Molluscum contagiosum is a poxvirus infection caused by direct skin contact. Sharing towels, baths or swimming pools with affected children may result in spread of the virus. Sexual transmission is the more likely route in the adolescent population. The lesions may become itchy because of surrounding eczema. Scratching can result in autoinoculation, as the mollusca spread along the skin in the direction of the scratching finger, occasionally producing linear lesions. Parents should be reassured that treatment is not required and the lesions will eventually settle on their own, usually without scarring. However, parents occasionally insist on treatment, particularly if the lesions increase in number. A large-bore needle may be used to puncture the lesion. Alternatively, if the child is able to tolerate it, cryotherapy may be attempted.

24   a and d

Vascular naevi may be divided into haemangiomas or vascular malformations. Haemangiomas are benign proliferative tumours of endothelial cells that are not usually present at birth. They usually appear after the first few weeks of birth. However, a pale patch may be noticed at birth at the site of their subsequent appearance. They are fast growing, with the bulk of growth occurring in the first 6 months of life. The rate of growth then slows down and usually no signs of enlargement are seen after the first year of life. Over time they involute and in the majority of cases they are fully resolved by the tenth birthday. Management is largely determined by their location. The vast majority of lesions do not require treatment and are managed by watchful waiting. There is a risk of them bleeding if caught and usual haemostatic measures should be taken if this occurs. Haemangiomas in the nappy area may ulcerate and hence require special attention with frequent applications of barrier creams. Exposed lesions should be protected from the sun with high-factor sun creams. Lesions around the eye (risk of amblyopia), mouth (feeding issues) and deep ones around the neck (tracheal compression) represent more serious manifestations that usually require more aggressive forms of treatment. Treatment options include steroids, laser therapy, propranolol and surgery. Licensed for use as migraine prophylaxis, propranolol is thought to cause vasoconstriction in the haemangioma, encourage cell death and prevent further angiogenesis (Starkey and Shahidullah, 2011). Sturge–Weber's syndrome is an association of a facial vascular malformation and a vascular malformation of the ipsilateral meninges and cerebral cortex. The capillary malformation occurs in the distribution of the first division of the trigeminal nerve. Vascular malformations by definition are fixed collections of dilated abnormal vessels (not proliferative like haemangiomas).

25 a

The canal of Schlemm is a circular canal responsible for draining the aqueous humour from the anterior chamber into the ciliary veins of the eye. Resistance of flow through the canal results in the build-up of pressure in the eye, leading to damage to the optic nerve. Congenital absence or abnormality of the canal (or any other congenital abnormality of the angle of the anterior chamber) can lead to primary buphthalmos or infantile glaucoma. The child will present with progressive enlargement of the eye as the intraocular pressure increases. The anterior chamber deepens and a progressive myopia may develop. Oedema, inflammation, photophobia and epiphoria usually ensue. Delayed diagnosis will invariably result in damage to the optic nerve head, leading to an irreversible reduction in vision. Treatment is by surgery and involves a trabeculectomy to allow increased drainage in the angle of the anterior chamber.

26 g

These are tough questions and are specifically designed to pick out the bright examination candidates. It is not uncommon to encounter the odd such question in the Diploma in Child Health exam that many primary care physicians may consider taking. Paediatric eponymous syndromes are many, and in most cases obscure, making it difficult to prepare for all eventual connotations such a question may take. In practical terms, knowledge of individual rare syndromes is rarely useful. The important point is that the physician is able to tell that something is wrong. The diagnostic process for such rare syndromes may take weeks to months as further symptoms and signs develop and the child is put through many investigations by paediatricians and specialist paediatricians. Low serum copper levels are a feature of Wilson's disease and Menkes's syndrome (also known as Menkes's kinky hair syndrome; the alternative name almost certainly giving away the answer too easily). In Wilson's disease the primary damage (from build-up of copper possibly due to a defective transporter responsible for removing copper from cells) is to the liver and the central nervous system and it should be considered in any child with abnormal liver function tests. Neurological manifestations may include psychiatric symptoms or extrapyramidal signs such as rigidity or tremor.

27 c

This question is also meant to confuse and test the confidence of the candidate in what they have learnt. Glucose-6-phosphate dehydrogenase deficiency leads to reduced glutathione levels in red cells, making them prone to haemolysis. It is an X-linked disorder and symptoms may vary from none to acute haemolysis requiring exchange transfusion in the neonate. Treatment is avoidance of stressors that may trigger haemolysis, such as dietary factors (e.g. fava beans), drugs (e.g. quinolones) or severe infections. It is the most common enzyme deficiency in the world. Von Gierke's disease is caused by a deficiency in glucose-6-phosphatase. It is a glycogen storage disorder. The lack of the enzyme leads to the cells' inability to convert glucose-6-phosphate to glucose. Alternative metabolic pathways convert the glucose precursor to lactic acid, the build-up of which is possibly responsible for the resultant retarded growth and osteoporosis. The glucose-6-phosphate may also be converted back into glycogen, the build-up of which in the liver causes hepatomegaly. It is a rare disorder.

28 a

McArdle's syndrome is another glycogen storage disease, resulting in inefficient use of energy substrate in muscle due to muscle phosphorylase deficiency. Exercise results in cramp that tends to settle with a period of rest. Creatine kinase levels may be elevated. It is generally a benign disorder and may not even be picked up until later in adult life when the individual takes up strenuous exercise. No specific treatment exists but the patient should be advised to stop exercise on the onset of muscle cramps. Failure to do so may result in rhabdomyolysis, myoglobinuria and subsequent renal failure.

29 a and c

Congenital heart disease is an umbrella term, encompassing a large number of cardiac defects of varying extent and severity. It can be divided into acyanotic and cyanotic lesions, with the latter associated with a greater number of early deaths because of the lack of circulating oxygenated blood. The cause may be environmental, genetic or multifactorial. Infections (e.g. congenital rubella syndrome) and drugs (e.g. lithium, alcohol) during pregnancy have been strongly linked with cardiac malformations. Ebstein's anomaly is a defect of the tricuspid valve and is very rare. A VSD is the commonest congenital heart lesion. In isolation it does not cause cyanosis. Usually VSDs are small and close spontaneously, mitigating the need for any surgery. However, if the VSD is large, increased pulmonary blood flow results in increased venous return to the left side of the heart, resulting in left atrial and ventricular enlargement. The right side of the heart may also enlarge as the left to right shunt increases, leading to increased blood flow into the pulmonary circulation and increased vascular resistance. It may take a few weeks for symptoms of a large VSD to develop, as the pulmonary resistance at birth is high, resulting in minimal shunting across the ventricular defect. The infant may present with dyspnoea, sweating when feeding, failure to thrive and recurrent respiratory infections. Dextrocardia does not automatically imply a defect in the heart anatomy. Tetralogy of Fallot is the commonest of the cyanotic congenital heart lesions. The 'tetralogy' consists of a VSD, pulmonary stenosis, an aorta overriding the ventricular septum and hypertrophy of the right ventricle. The presentation of Fallot's tetralogy depends largely on the extent and severity of the aforementioned abnormalities, primarily the degree of right ventricular outflow obstruction. Usually the infant is not cyanosed at birth and this develops later in life. In the most severe form of Fallot's tetralogy, pulmonary atresia with VSD, the infant will be cyanosed shortly after birth and may be completely dependent on a patent ductus arteriosus for survival.

30   b

Chest pain in the paediatric population is a common presenting symptom in general practice but it is rarely serious. Musculoskeletal pain arising from ribs, muscles and other structures in the thoracic area is common. The usual concern is cardiac chest pain due to well-publicised campaigns concerning adults. Cardiac problems rarely cause chest pain in healthy children, although consideration must be given to arrhythmias, congenital heart problems and inflammatory (e.g. pericarditis) conditions. Pericarditis classically produces a sharp pain that is worse with coughing, deep breathing and leaning forwards. The child is usually not very well either. Tietze's syndrome is caused by a single (most commonly second or third), swollen and painful costochondral junction (hence differing from costochondritis, which involves multiple costochondral junctions that are not swollen). The diagnosis is clinical and the condition is self-limiting, settling over the course of a few weeks to months. The underlying cause is unclear but a preceding viral infection may be responsible. Slipping rib syndrome is caused by a disruption in the fibrous tissue joining the eighth, ninth and tenth ribs. This may be through trauma or lifting resulting in the costal cartilages impinging on the intercostal nerves. Pulling the lower costal cartilages forwards reproduces the pain, allowing the diagnosis to be made. However, abdominal causes of the pain may need to be ruled out to ascertain diagnostic certainty. The pain may last many months. Texidor's twinge, or precordial catch syndrome, is common in children and adolescents. A sharp pain, of short duration, occurs mostly just under the left breast or nipple. The pain may be made worse with deep inspiration (though others find relief with a deep breath) and may occur a few times a day. It does not signify any underlying problem and may be due to an impinged intercostal nerve or even associated with anxiety. No treatment is required and it tends to self-resolve (Ives, *et al.*, 2010).

31   e

Deficiency in niacin (vitamin B_3) causes pellagra, which classically causes the triad of dementia, diarrhoea and dermatitis (Hendricks, 1991) – the dermatitis being the most common manifestation in children. Niacin is a water-soluble vitamin and is derived from the diet and from the conversion of the amino acid tryptophan. Bioavailability is high in meat and fortified grains. The dermatitis of pellagra affects exposed areas such as the neck (Casal's necklace, named after the Spanish physician who first described the rash in peasants), cheeks and the extremities and may mimic sunburn. It is common in parts of the world where the main food source is maize, because of the lack of bioavailability of niacin and tryptophan in maize. Other causes include use of the anti-tuberculosis drug isoniazid (which blocks tryptophan conversion to niacin), carcinoid tumour (which diverts tryptophan conversion to serotonin) and Hartnup disease (impaired tryptophan transport).

32   c

Infantile beriberi is caused by vitamin B_1 (thiamine) deficiency and is associated with a predominantly polished rice diet (the outer layer, which is rich in the vitamin, is removed due to over-soaking or washing the rice). The thiamine-deficient mum suckles the child with thiamine-deficient milk. The young infant may be irritable and drowsy in the early stages, only to later present with acute cardiac failure. Neurological manifestations of the disease include encephalopathy, seizures, coma and eventually death. Treatment is with parental thiamine administration. Resolution of the symptoms confirms the diagnosis.

33   f

Once the scourge of seafarers (earning it the name *the plague of the sea*), scurvy, as a result of vitamin C deficiency, is now rare. Vitamin C plays important and varied functions in the body and hence the signs and symptoms of deficiency may also be wide and varied. Petechial skin haemorrhages, irritability and impaired growth may be early signs seen in childhood. Bleeding gums due to fragile capillaries may result in loosening of the newly erupting teeth. Bleeding may occur around bones, leading to painful swellings of the lower limbs. Treatment is with vitamin C replacement.

Other manifestations of this exam question could have included xerophthalmia (vitamin A deficiency), rickets (vitamin D deficiency), acrodermatitis enteropathica (zinc deficiency) and Keshan disease (selenium deficiency).

34   b and d

Protein-energy malnutrition encompasses a number of conditions of which kwashiorkor and marasmus are the best described. Marasmus is essentially caused by a low-calorific diet in which the child has access to very little of what is otherwise a nutritionally complete diet. The child is usually ravenous (unlike the child with kwashiorkor who is listless, irritable and has a depressed appetite). Biochemical abnormalities are less common in marasmus in comparison to kwashiorkor. The child is thin with reduced weight and loss of fat and muscle tissue. Provision of ample calories results in the child regaining weight and the prognosis is generally good when identified and treated in infancy. Kwashiorkor is caused by a deficiency in protein intake that occurs as breast milk is eliminated from the diet. Low protein content of the weaned foods leads to a decrease in total energy intake and nutritional deficiencies. Concurrent increase in risk of enteric infections from various bacteria worsens the nutritional deficiencies and increases the risk of death. Although more common in the developing world, protein-energy malnutrition is seen in the industrialised world in the context of neglect and fad diets.

35 c

These are all syndromes associated with mental retardation. Prader–Willi's syndrome is an autosomal dominant genetic condition in which the child may be hypotonic with developmental delay and have behavioural issues, specifically concerning food. Obesity is common and may not be entirely down to overeating, as minor endocrine abnormalities are likely to contribute to the problem. Hypogonadism is also a common feature. Genetic testing is required for the diagnosis. Angelman's syndrome is also known as happy puppet syndrome and has been discussed elsewhere. Rubella syndrome is caused by foetal infection with rubella in non-immune mothers in the first trimester. This is a particularly devastating infection, leading to a number of mental and physical handicaps including deafness, visual problems and microcephaly. Down's syndrome is also associated with obesity.

36 f

Abnormal development of the third and fourth pharyngeal arches during embryonic development results in DiGeorge's syndrome. The majority of cases are caused by chromosomal deletion at 22q11, although other chromosomal abnormalities have also been implicated. It results in immunodeficiency (due to inadequate thymic development), congenital heart defects, hypocalcaemia (due to underactive parathyroids) and abnormal facies. An extra copy of chromosome 18 results in Edwards's syndrome, in which there may be a wide variety of congenital defects and mental retardation. Trisomy 21 is commonly known as Down's syndrome.

37 g

Lyme disease is caused by the spirochete bacterium *Borrelia burgdorferi*. *B. burgdorferi* is transferred to humans via the hard tick *Ixodes dammini*, which feeds on animals infected with the bacterium. Introduction of the bacterium into the human bloodstream via tick saliva occurs during a tick bite. Patients may recall this tick bite and the resultant macular lesion that appears at the site of the bite. This lesion then expands over the course of a week and develops into the characteristic rash of Lyme disease: erythema chronicum migrans. While this is occurring the patient may suffer from a prodromal phase in which there is fever and general malaise. The appearance of the typical rash should raise suspicions and trigger appropriate investigations that may include serology (to look for antibodies against the bacterium) and culture from appropriate fluid or tissue. Untreated, there is a significant risk of developing the late manifestations of Lyme disease, which include neurological abnormalities (e.g. meningitis, cranial neuropathy, peripheral neuropathy), heart disease (e.g. myocarditis, pericarditis, atrioventricular block) and rheumatological disease such as arthritis and fatigue. Rarely, the eyes, liver, spleen and testicles may also be involved. Doxycycline is the first-choice antibiotic. Summer forest walkers should be advised to cover up well and remove attached ticks promptly. Q fever is another bacterial zoonosis caused by the bacterium *Coxiella burnetii*.

38 d

Congenital adrenal hyperplasia is a group of disorders inherited in an autosomal recessive pattern. They are characterised by abnormal adrenal corticosteroid production due to a deficiency in one of five enzymes involved in their production. A 21-hydroxylase deficiency accounts for the commonest form of CAH, leading to cortisol deficiency with or without aldosterone deficiency. The resultant increase in adrenocorticotrophic hormone stimulates hyperplasia of the adrenal glands. Since cortisol production is defective, its precursors, in the form of adrenal androgens, poor out into the bloodstream causing virilisation in the child. In girls this may cause enlargement of the clitoris to the point that she may be mistaken for a normal male. Internal organ development is normal. Diagnosis in boys is usually in early childhood, as there is abnormal enlargement of the penis and rapid growth. In the more severe form of CAH (salt-wasting form), the zona glomerulosa of the kidney is also involved, resulting in loss of urinary sodium. The child will present with dehydration, vomiting and shock.

39 a, b, d and e

H. pylori is a slow-growing bacterium that has been linked frequently with stomach problems such as gastric ulcers and chronic gastritis. It has been shown also to increase the risk of developing gastric cancer. However, most people infected with *H. pylori* are, and remain, asymptomatic. Investigations for infection are not indicated in children presenting with functional abdominal pain. In the child, the primary objective should always be to diagnose the underlying condition causing the problem. Simply attempting to detect *H. pylori* infection is needless and can be distracting, as all the symptoms may wrongly be attributed to the bacterium. This may then lead the child through unnecessary investigations, some of which are invasive. Hence routine testing in general practice is not recommended. Testing children with unexplained iron-deficiency anaemia or who have first-degree relatives with gastric cancer is considered acceptable because of the demonstrated links between these conditions and the bacterium. Endoscopy and positive biopsy culture (or positive histopathology) is the referenced standard of diagnosis at present. Urea breath tests and stool antigen testing for *H. pylori* are both recognised and accepted, non-invasive methods of diagnosing the infection. Serological tests for *H. pylori* have variable sensitivities and specificities and are considered inaccurate, restricting their use to epidemiological studies only (Crowley, *et al.*, 2012).

40   b

The acronym HOP helps remember the presenting features of nephrotic syndrome. The triad of **h**ypoalbuminaemia (and hyperlipidaemia), **o**edema and **p**roteinuria indicate the presence of nephrotic syndrome. In children it is caused mainly by two idiopathic diseases: (1) minimal change nephrotic syndrome and (2) focal segmental glomerulosclerosis. An increased risk of infectious complications among children with nephrotic syndrome has long been recognised. Cellulitis and spontaneous bacterial peritonitis are not too infrequent complications of nephrotic syndrome and one should be on guard against their development. Children should receive pneumococcal vaccination. Overwhelming bacterial infection in nephrotic syndrome still carries a significant mortality rate and hence should not be taken lightly when seen in primary care. Thromboembolic complications are also more common in nephrotic syndrome because of the hypercoagulable state it encourages. They are, however, less common in children than in adults. Hyperlipidaemia, hypertension, hypercoagulability and use of steroids as treatment all increase the cardiovascular risk in sufferers of nephrotic syndrome. Vitamin D deficiency due to loss of vitamin D–binding protein through the kidney may lead to secondary hyperparathyroidism. Progression to end-stage renal disease may be inevitable for some children who end up requiring dialysis. Children who respond to steroids will tend to have the best long-term prognosis.

41 c

Pes planus or flat feet in children is usually part of normal feet development, particularly in the newly weight-bearing infant. The longitudinal arch of the foot is flat. Associated changes seen include valgus eversion of the heel and outward turning of the forefoot. Laxity at the knee joint resulting in genu valgum may also be present. The child should be encouraged to walk around the room while these changes are observed. Asking an older child to stand on tiptoe may reveal an underlying normal arch. A degree of ligamentous laxity on examination of the heel is expected and probably responsible for the heel eversion. In such benign cases, parents should be reassured and advised that a normal arch is expected to develop with time. Appropriate footwear, walking barefoot and foot inversion exercises (encouraging the child to pick things with his or her feet) may all be encouraged. The child, however, should be monitored for the development of red flags that include pain, hypermobility or rigidity. This may be due to bony or soft tissue abnormalities leading to 'tarsal coalition', a congenitally vertical talus (rocker-bottom feet) or neurological problems such as cerebral palsy.

42 g

Pectus carinatum or pigeon chest is thought to be caused by defective growth of the costal cartilages at the junction of the ribs with the sternum. This is usually not associated with any functional defect. However, it may be a cause of psychological distress to the child and the parents. Parents should be reassured that the development of breasts and chest muscles will gradually make the chest appear more cosmetically acceptable. Some children, however, may complain of reduced exercise tolerance as a result of the deformity and hence lung function tests may be of use. Some centres promote the use of a chest brace; however, their usefulness is unclear. Severe cases may be treated with surgery. There is likely to be a high incidence of parental anxiety and it is usually appropriate to refer to a suitable specialist so that all the available options may be discussed. Pectus excavatum (funnel chest) is almost the opposite deformity, as the sternum is depressed.

43   d

Blount's disease or infantile tibia vara is a knee condition caused by abnormal development of the upper tibial growth plate, usually on the medial aspect. The underlying cause is unknown but abnormal pressures on the developing growth plate may be responsible. This results in beaking of the growth plate, felt as a bony mass in the child in the case outlined here. With time the tibia becomes internally rotated and angulates medially. It may be initially difficult to differentiate from physiological bowing of the knees (genu varum). However, in Blount's disease the abnormality will continue to worsen, in contrast to the spontaneous resolution seen with genu varum. Treatment options include braces and surgery.

44   a, c and e

Autism forms part of a whole spectrum of developmental disorders that are termed as the autistic spectrum disorders (ASDs). The main three clinical features are:
- impaired social relationships
- language abnormalities
- ritualistic and compulsive behaviours.

The extent of impairment in these categories determines where the child lies on the spectrum. Autism represents the more severe form of ASD in that the impairments in these categories are significant. Parents will often tell of how the child smiles little, lacks appropriate responses to emotional cues such as hugging, demonstrates poor eye-to-eye contact and difficulty in forming friendships and appropriate social relationships and interactions. Language development may also be very impaired with some children not developing language at all. Repetition of words or phrases (echolalia) is another feature of impaired language development in autistic children. Comprehension is also usually affected. Ritualistic play and obsessions with odd objects may be manifested with the child becoming agitated with any change in their set routine or environment. Learning disability and low intelligence may co-exist in autism, which usually impacts their ability to live independent lives in the future. Asperger's syndrome represents a milder form of the ASD in which language development is not so severely affected. A third category, 'pervasive developmental disorder not otherwise specified', is used to describe children who fall in the middle of the aforementioned two categories. Maternal sodium valproate use in pregnancy and a gestational age of less than 35 weeks is associated with an increased prevalence of autism. Treatment is centred on promoting as much normal development as possible. The provision of support to the family is as important as providing the various available therapies to the child.

45 c

All of the answers in this question are associated with sensorineural deafness. Waardenburg's syndrome is associated with skull and facial abnormalities with deafness. In Usher's syndrome the deafness is associated with retinitis pigmentosa and visual field defects. Retinitis pigmentosa may also be present in Refsum's syndrome, along with night blindness and mental retardation. Spinal deformities and deafness are a feature of Klippel–Feil's syndrome. These hereditary causes of prenatal deafness are thankfully rare. Prenatal exposure to viruses (e.g. cytomegalovirus, toxoplasmosis) and drugs (e.g. gentamicin) may also cause sensorineural deafness in the child. Postnatally, measles, mumps and meningococcal or pneumococcal meningitis may cause sensorineural deafness.

46 e

This child is presenting with a typical history of migraine preceded by a visual aura. The headache is thought to be due to vasodilation and increased blood flow to the extracranial vessels. Corresponding vasoconstriction of various intracranial vessels produces the varied neurological features of migraine. A history of migraine in a close family member pretty much nails the diagnosis when the clinical presentation is typical of migraine. In such cases, when neurological examination is also normal, further investigation is rarely necessary. Occasionally, to quell parental anxiety, brain imaging may be required. In this case, where there is little doubt about the diagnosis, of the options listed, prophylactic medicine to prevent attacks is the most appropriate next step. Prophylactic agents include β-blockers, pizotifen and the tricylic antidepressant amitriptylline. Further investigations are warranted where the diagnosis is in doubt or abnormal neurology is elicited. Keeping a food diary can be extremely helpful in identifying potential triggers of migraine and hence limiting attacks without medication. The combined oral contraceptive would be absolutely contraindicated in this case.

47   a

The history of headache in this child sounds quite benign. Usually, it is the parents who are more concerned by the child occasionally mentioning that his or her head hurts. There are no worrying features in the history that would point towards serious pathology. A full neurological (including fundoscopy) examination should be performed. If everything appears normal it is appropriate to suggest to the parents that this may be an ocular headache caused by a refraction error and the child should have an eye test. Whether refractive errors actually cause headaches is somewhat controversial. However, one study (Gil-Gouveia and Martins, 2002) found that adequate correction of refractive errors in children who suffered with headaches (and had refractive errors) resulted in improvement in symptoms in 72.5% of children. Thirty-eight per cent of children reported a complete remission of headache, suggesting the possibility of a causal link. The child should be encouraged to drink more water. At this point, if adequately reassured, the parents will ask you whether the headache is to do with the amount of video games the child plays. At this point a 'wise, non-committing nod' may just allow the parents to tell the child to take note that the doctor thinks that he or she should spend less time playing video games!

48   f

This history is suggestive of cluster headaches, a thankfully rare phenomenon in children. As the name suggests, the intense one-sided headaches occur in clusters over a certain period of time, usually lasting a few hours. Patients may present with extreme restlessness and intense headache, enough to cause some to bang their heads against the walls of the casualty department. Autonomic features such as redness, watering and swelling of the eye, sweating of the face and nasal blockage may occur. Simple analgesics are generally not effective but are usually given. This child will require brain imaging to rule out secondary causes of headache. However, in the first instance the most appropriate step is to try to relieve the pain. Treatment options include 100% oxygen, methysergide, triptans and ergotamine (Majumdar, *et al.*, 2008).

49   b and d

Hodgkin's lymphoma most commonly affects the cervical and supraclavicular glands, although mediastinal involvement may be seen in two-thirds of children with the disease. An increased risk is seen in children from higher socio-economic groups. Diagnosis is made by taking a biopsy from the affected node, which may feel firm or rubbery. The cell that is affected in Hodgkin's disease is the Reed–Sternberg cell. Although a diagnosis of Hodgkin's lymphoma cannot be made in the absence of Reed–Sternberg cells, they are not pathognomonic for the disease, as they may also be present in some non-Hodgkin's lymphomas and Epstein–Barr virus infection. The Ann Arbor staging system is used to help stage the disease. Stage I denotes involvement of a single lymph node region whereas stage IV represents diffuse involvement of extralymphatic organs or tissues. The staging may be suffixed with A or B. The suffix 'B' denotes presence of B symptoms: fever, night sweats or greater than 10% weight loss in the preceding 6 months and is associated with a worse prognosis. The suffix 'A' is designated in the absence of these symptoms. Chemotherapy forms the mainstay of treatment although radiotherapy is also needed at times.

50   a

Haemophilia A, also known as classical haemophilia, is among the commonest of the bleeding disorders and is caused by an absence or low levels of factor VIIIc. Haemophilia B, or Christmas disease, is caused by a deficiency of factor IX. The two conditions present in a similar fashion clinically. Both are X-linked recessive disorders and a good family history enables a diagnosis to be made. Unexplained bruising and haemarthrosis, when the child is mobile, occasionally raise concerns regarding non-accidental injury. Von Willebrand's disease is caused by a deficiency or abnormal function of von Willebrand factor and its most common form is inherited in autosomal dominant fashion. Epistaxis can be a recurring problem in this condition. Idiopathic thrombocytopaenic purpura is the commonest of the immune thrombocytopaenias in which there is an increased destruction of platelets. Bernard–Soulier's syndrome is a congenital disorder in which there is a failure of platelet production.

51   h

Mumps is a notifiable disease and may present in a non-specific fashion, like other viral infections, with fever and malaise resulting in the correct diagnosis not being made. The incubation period for mumps is between 14 and 21 days. Involvement of the parotid glands is what makes it easily recognisable, particularly when the swelling is impressive resulting in the angle of the jaw becoming impalpable. The swelling may be unilateral to start with, progressing to become bilateral in the majority of cases. Mumps can affect any organ in the body and hence multiple symptoms may be seen. However, involvement of the central nervous system (aseptic meningitis), testicles (orchitis) and pancreas (pancreatitis) certainly raise the suspicion of mumps, particularly if there is unappreciable swelling of the parotid glands. Diagnosis may be confirmed by demonstration of rise in antibody titres or direct culturing of the virus. Treatment is usually supportive and includes rest, plenty of fluids to keep the mouth moist and clean (as it may become dry as a result of swelling of the salivary gland ducts), analgesia and support and ice bags for painful testis. Boys (and their parents) should be reassured that sterility is rare, even after severe orchitis.

52   a

This child has hand, foot and mouth disease caused, in the majority of cases, by Coxsackie virus A16. Other strains of Coxsackie group A virus have also been implicated in outbreaks of the illness. The child is usually only mildly unwell and the main concern may be the appearance of the vesicles or reluctance to eat and drink due to the lesions inside the mouth. Serious complications are extremely rare and in most cases all symptoms will have settled in a week. Because of the mild nature of the majority of cases, there is no need to keep the child off school.

53   d

This is the typical presentation of roseola infantum. Other names for this condition include sixth disease (a historical reference to the six rash-causing illnesses of childhood), exanthema subitum and 3-day fever. The rash appears as the child improves in his or her condition and most parents will tell you that they would not have come to see you had the rash not appeared. Parvovirus B19 causes slapped cheek syndrome, also known as fifth disease.

54 a, b and c

This question introduces the fascinating concept of the non-specific effects of vaccines. This refers to the holistic effect of the vaccine on the body, including on organisms not intended by the vaccine. This is an area of growing interest, with the World Health Organization setting up a group of experts to look into this specific area of vaccine effect as recently as March 2013 (*see* WHO, 2013). It is no longer possible to look at vaccines simply modulating immunological response against the intended organism only. The way the vaccine interacts with the immune system is modulated by previous infections and immunisations. The bacillus Calmette–Guérin vaccine has been shown to reduce mortality from diseases other than tuberculosis by up to 25%. The sequence in which vaccines are given is also important. The increased mortality associated with the diphtheria, tetanus and pertussis vaccine appears to be reversed by a subsequent dose of measles vaccine. A greater amount of research in this field is likely to yield a fascinating insight into how vaccines interplay with other organisms and the immune system. Option d is false, as maternal immunisation with pertussis is currently being recommended between 28 and 38 weeks of pregnancy. Option e (known as cocooning strategy) has been shown to be effective, albeit difficult to implement.

55 d

Vaccines may be live attenuated, inactivated, polysaccharide vaccines or genetically engineered. Attenuation of a live organism refers to weakening it in a laboratory before using it to stimulate active immunity in the recipient. Usually only one dose is required, as they stimulate a more effective immune response in the recipient. However, second doses are needed for some vaccinations (e.g. measles, mumps and rubella) where a sufficient response is not mounted in all individuals after the first dose. Inactivated vaccines require multiple doses where the first dose merely primes the immune system, with an effective immune response mounted on subsequent doses. Oral polio vaccine (the Sabin vaccine) is live, but in the UK injectable polio (the Salk vaccine) is used, which is inactivated. Rotavirus vaccine has been recently introduced into the routine immunisation schedule in the UK, given at 2 and 3 months of age.

56   d

This scenario describes labial adhesions, a not too uncommon scenario in young girls. The adhesions start from the posterior vulva and may extend across its entirety until only the urethral meatus is the visible structure. Differentiating between labial adhesions and congenital vaginal agenesis is important. The underlying cause is not always clear but it is likely to be due to local irritation resulting in fusion of the labial folds. Treatment of adhesions is not always necessary, as the problem may resolve spontaneously as the child reaches puberty and produces endogenous oestrogen. However, this child seems to be affected by the problem and hence a small amount of oestrogen cream applied twice a day for 2 weeks is indicated. This will usually resolve the problem without the need for further courses. Genital hygiene and salt baths are recommended to prevent further episodes of localised irritation leading to a recurrence of the problem. Surgery is very rarely needed. Podophyllotoxin is used in the treatment of genital warts.

57   a

Threadworm infections are common in young children. It may cause no symptoms whatsoever, although anal itching (due to deposition of eggs) is the most common presentation. In girls they may be a cause of vulval and vaginal irritation. Whether they are responsible for undiagnosed cases of abdominal pain or wrongly suspected appendicitis is unlikely. Eggs are picked up from anal scratching or from contaminated bedding, and ingested. The eggs hatch in the upper bowel and the larvae mature into adult worms in the caecum. Eggs are again laid on the perianal skin and the cycle continues. Eggs trapped in nails (which are then bitten) result in repetition of the life cycle of the worm. A single dose of mebendazole 100 mg has a greater than 90% success rate. The dose should be repeated after 2 weeks. Advise the parents to regularly wash the child's hands before meals and after visits to the toilet. An early-morning bath or rinse of the anal area helps clear any eggs that may have been laid in the night.

58   i

Koplik's spots are pathognomonic of measles. They may be difficult to spot, and disappear as the illness progresses. There have been recent outbreaks of measles due to a lack of uptake of the measles, mumps and rubella vaccine in the last decade, because of unfounded fears of its link with autism. The child is usually very unwell and irritable with a high-grade fever. There is a high complication rate and may involve the lungs, eyes, ears, central nervous system and gastrointestinal tract. Subacute sclerosing panencephalitis is a rare complication of measles in which the virus survives in the cerebrum, only to be reactivated years later. It presents with behavioural change and a drop in intellectual level. This then progresses to movement disorders and mental deterioration. Severe dementia, seizures and eventually coma may follow.

59   a and e

Differentiating between T1DM and T2DM is not always straightforward. However, in the case of a child presenting with DKA, the differentiation is of secondary importance. The first priority is to start insulin and rehydrate the patient in order to reduce the blood glucose level. With trends in obesity increasing in childhood, T2DM is set to become a major health issue in this population. When diagnosed early, efforts should be made to distinguish between the two types of diabetes. A normal or high level of insulin and C-peptide is suggestive of T2DM, as is a positive family history, increased body mass index and lack of antibodies associated with T1DM. Children with T2DM presenting with severe hyperglycaemia and ketosis should also be initiated on insulin, at least for a short period to allow better glycaemic control. This is also likely to instil understanding of the seriousness of the illness and hopefully better compliance with the lifestyle modifications and oral anti-diabetic medication. Evidence for effectiveness of lifestyle modifications alone is poor and hence many would argue that metformin is started concomitantly at the time of diagnosis. Children and their families should be offered dietetic support upon diagnosis and encouraged to take regular exercise (Copeland, *et al.*, 2013).

60   d

Beckwith–Wiedemann's syndrome is associated with tall stature, whereas the rest are all associated with short stature. Any chronic disease such as cystic fibrosis, Crohn's disease and asthma may be a cause for short stature. Other causes of short stature include dysmorphic syndromes, nutritional deficiencies, low birthweight due to intrauterine growth restriction, skeletal dysplasias such as achondroplasia, familial short stature (due to short parents), psychosocial deprivation and constitutional delay of growth and puberty. Hormonal causes of short stature include growth hormone deficiency or insufficiency, hypothyroidism and Cushing's syndrome. In the absence of a cause, idiopathic short stature is diagnosed. The use of growth hormone in the treatment of idiopathic short stature has been a contentious issue, with some considering it to be a punishment for short stature, arguing, with some merit, that we should help the child in acquiring important coping skills to deal with their shorter stature (Brook, 1997). A reasonable start would be to not 'medicalise' idiopathic short stature and reassure the child and his or her parents that the child is normal. However, studies have shown that growth hormone administration in children with idiopathic short stature is effective in partially reducing the height deficit as an adult, albeit not by a huge amount (Deodati and Cianfarani, 2011). One may often find oneself in a situation where well-informed parents will demand growth hormone in such cases to maximise the growth potential of their child. The potential risk of cancer and the stigmatisation of an otherwise normal child should be considered before prescribing growth hormone in such cases. One is also duty bound to contemplate the ethical considerations of 'cosmetic' growth hormone administration in a cash-strapped National Health Service.

61   d

Alagille's syndrome is an autosomal dominant disorder in which there is paucity of the intrahepatic bile ducts. The resultant chronic cholestasis causes jaundice, pruritis and hypercholesterolemia. Dysmorphic faces, cardiac anomalies, vertebral anomalies, failure to thrive and developmental delay are features of the syndrome. Budd–Chiari's syndrome is a rare condition in which there is obstruction of the hepatic veins. Gilbert's syndrome is a usually harmless condition in which reduced levels of a particular enzyme (uridine-diphosphate glucuronosyltransferase) in the liver results in slightly raised serum bilirubin levels. Criggler–Najjar's syndrome is a rare disorder in which a defective enzyme results in defective breakdown of bile, causing its levels to rise.

62   e

Biliary atresia is a disease of unknown cause in which there is inflammatory obstruction and destruction of the intra- and extrahepatic bile ducts. It is the most common cause of neonatal liver disease. Early identification is necessary for the neonate to have the best chance of recovery. Kasai portoenterostomy is effective in achieving good biliary drainage, thus improving the chances of the neonate reaching adolescence without the need for a liver transplantation. It should be suspected in all neonates with prolonged jaundice, raised conjugated bilirubin level and pale stools, triggering an urgent referral to a paediatrician.

63   i

Although lung manifestations are more common with cystic fibrosis, it remains a rare but important cause of prolonged neonatal jaundice. The salty taste on kissing the child forms the basis of the sweat test. Excessive salt loss in the sweat of a child suffering from cystic fibrosis is demonstrated by passing a weak electrical current into the skin to induce sweating. The levels of sodium and chloride are then measured in the sweat.

64   b and c

The Apgar score is widely used to assess birth asphyxia. It has the advantage of being reasonably objective with a documented score of 0–10, usually measured at 1 and 5 minutes after birth. Five (not four) variables are measured:

- *heart rate* (0 if absent, 1 if <100 beats/min, 2 if >100 beats/min)
- *respiratory effort* (0 if absent, 1 for weak cry, 2 for strong cry)
- *muscle tone* (0 if limp, 1 if some flexion is present, 2 for good flexion)
- *reflex irritability in response to a form of stimulus* (0 if no response, 1 for a grimace, 2 for a cry)
- *colour of child* (0 if pale and generally cyanosed, 1 if centrally pink and peripherally cyanosed, 2 for being pink).

It is immediately obvious that the test is not completely objective, as the difference between a weak and strong cry or level of flexion may be subtle. Also assessing the degree of cyanosis in dark-skinned infants cannot be scored on level of 'pinkness'. Nonetheless, it still allows for the documentation of a quantifiable score immediately after birth. Prematurity, maternal medication, cardiovascular and neurological conditions of the newborn will adversely affect the Apgar scores with or without any significant asphyxia. Despite the fact that a very low Apgar score (3 and below) is directly related to an increased risk of death in a full-term infant, it is generally poorly predictive of long-term outcomes. Nelson and Ellenberg (1981) recorded Apgar scores for 49 000 infants. They found that a large proportion of children developing cerebral palsy later in life scored reasonably well, with 55% having scores of 7–10 at 1 minute and 73% scoring 7–10 at 5 minutes.

65   e

Reye's syndrome is a rare form of encephalopathy that is frequently fatal. Disturbance in the structure and function of mitochondria seems to be the underlying problem, which leads to a devastatingly acute onset of illness. The underlying cause seems to be unknown but aspirin has been linked with its development, as has a preceding viral infection. The child presents with vomiting and features of encephalopathy. Biochemical evidence of liver involvement further raises the suspicion. Mortality rates are as high as 40%, with a significant proportion of survivors suffering permanent brain injury. Many inborn errors of metabolism (IEMs) present similarly to Reye's syndrome. Increasing understanding of the cellular and molecular dysfunctions of IEMs has resulted in fewer cases of Reye's syndrome being diagnosed (Schrör, 2007). Whether this is due to a successful public health campaign to reduce the use of aspirin in children or better understanding of IEMs is anyone's guess. The Medicines and Healthcare Products Regulatory Agency has issued precautionary advice to avoid the use of salicylate-containing oral gels (such as Bonjela) in children under the age of 16.

66   d

Haematocolpos is a rare condition caused by the onset of menstruation with an imperforate hymen. Blood accumulates in the vagina and may eventually cause swelling of the uterus and even the fallopian tubes. This may manifest itself as a mass, which may extend into the pelvis and be felt transabdominally. Urinary hesitancy and frequency due to pressure from the mass may follow. Dissection of the membrane under general anaesthetic results in a release of the collected blood and subsequent relief from the symptoms. Wilkie's syndrome is a rare syndrome that may cause acute or chronic abdominal pain in children and adults. The third part of the duodenum is compressed between the superior mesenteric artery and the aorta, resulting in symptoms of upper gastrointestinal obstruction.

67   a

Intussusception refers to the herniation of the intestine into itself. Part of the bowel serves as the apex from where the herniation begins. The exact cause is unknown but it has been linked with viral infections. The virus causes inflammation of lymphoid tissue in the bowel (Peyer's patch). The swollen, enlarged part of the bowel then invaginates into the colon for a variable distance, presenting itself at the anus in the most severe of cases. Since it is commonest in infants between the ages of 3 and 9 months, the change in bowel flora as a result of weaning may have a causative role. Ultimately, pressure of the herniated bowel against the wall of normal bowel causes colicky abdominal pain that worsens as the condition progresses. Vomiting commonly follows. Redcurrant jelly stool is frequently associated with intussusceptions and is stool mixed with mucus and blood. Treatment involves attempting to reduce the herniating bowel by means of passing an air enema. Surgery is required if this fails.

68   c

Pyloric stenosis usually presents in the first few weeks of life as parents report an increasing frequency of vomiting. A congenitally thickened pylorus results in obstruction of outflow of stomach contents. As the condition progresses, projectile vomiting follows, as the vomit no longer trickles down the front of the infant but rather shoots over the shoulder of the anxious parent. The vomitus may become progressively blood stained because of the resulting gastritis. The infant usually feels hungry after vomiting and is keen to feed again. Traditionally the diagnosis is made during examination of the child after a test feed. The physician is able to feel the olive-shaped mass in the right hypochondrium. Peristalsis may be visible as the surrounding muscles contract to push the feed beyond the narrowing. The loss of gastric acid as a result of vomiting leads to hypochloraemia, alkalosis and hypokalaemia. However, pyloric stenosis is usually diagnosed before the classical biochemical hallmarks develop, because of early suspicion and use of ultrasound scanning (Hulka, *et al.*, 1997). Treatment involves a pyloromyotomy, which may be performed laparoscopically.

69   a and c

Male infant circumcision can be an emotive topic. For some it is a religious right and duty, the practice of which goes back thousands of years. For others it is an assault on a non-consenting child and a breach of the child's human rights. This question, thankfully, is more about objective scientific evidence regarding the benefits and harms of circumcision rather than the ethical and moral dilemmas surrounding it. The overall consensus of scientific evidence seems to be towards greater health benefits compared with the small risks associated with the procedure. Indeed, the American Academy of Pediatrics issued an update on their circumcision policy, stating that the increased health benefits warranted third-party payment for the procedure. This was received with some stiff opposition, mainly from various European medical associations. The American Academy of Pediatrics does not, however, recommend routine male infant circumcisions, leaving the decision mainly with the parents. Health benefits include a reduced risk of developing HIV in areas of high HIV prevalence such as Africa. Circumcision is also likely to be protective against syphilis, human papillomavirus and genital herpes. A reduced risk of chlamydia and gonorrhoea has not been demonstrated. The abrasion and micro-tear-prone inner surface of the foreskin may be responsible for the increased risk of developing sexually transmitted infections. Circumcision is not associated with an increased risk of cervical cancer in the partner. On the contrary, it may be protective against its development. The risk of penile cancer is reduced with circumcision. Measuring sexual satisfaction, sensitivity and function is difficult; however, the literature does not suggest that circumcised males are at any disadvantage in these departments! Any such suggestions may be extrapolations of studies done on men who were circumcised as adults in whom reduced masturbatory pleasure and increased threshold for light-touch sensitivity has been demonstrated.

70   b

Wilms's tumour accounts for the majority of kidney tumours in the paediatric age group. It may present as part of WAGR syndrome – **W**ilms's tumour, **a**niridia (lack of iris), **g**enitourinary abnormalities and mental **r**etardation. A deletion on chromo-some 11 of a tumour suppressor gene, resulting in a loss of heterozygosity, is thought to be involved in the development of Wilms's tumour. Other syndromes with which Wilms's tumour has been associated with include Denys–Drash's syndrome (pseudohermaphroditism and renal failure) and Beckwith–Wiedemann's syndrome (macroglossia, organomegaly, macrosomia). It may be picked up as an asymptomatic abdominal mass in some children. Pain, non-specific malaise and haematuria may be the presenting symptoms in up to a third of children.

71   c

72   a

73   e

Perthes's disease is a self-limiting disorder in which there is ischaemia of the femoral head. It is more common in boys and usually has an insidious onset. As with all hip pathologies, the pain may be poorly localised, with the child complain-ing of knee or thigh pain. Destruction of the epiphyses (and sometimes of the adjacent metaphysis) interspersed with periods of reconstruction result in ana-tomical abnormalities of the femoral head and neck. Hip movements are reduced because of the anatomical abnormalities and protective muscle spasm. FBC, ESR and CRP are normal. Being able to correctly diagnose septic arthritis is of the utmost importance because of the potential of devastating joint destruction. Large joints are mainly affected. Distinguishing septic arthritis from transient synovitis of the hip can be quite challenging. The presence of fever, raised CRP, raised ESR, a raised serum white cell count and inability to weight-bear all suggest septic arthritis (Caird, *et al.*, 2006). The child is usually unwell. Slipped upper femoral epiphysis is commoner in boys who are obese and gonadally immature. Gradual slippage of the capital femoral epiphyses posteriorly and inferiorly results in pain, swelling and reduction in hip movements. This is usually a slow process. The boy in Question 73 has developed acute slipped upper femoral epiphysis in which the twisting injury has caused an acute slip of the capital femoral epiphyses. This may be amenable to reduction by gentle manipulation and pinning. Reduction in a chronic slip is avoided because of the potential of compromising the blood supply to the femoral head. Bone tumours can present with night pain or as pathological fractures. Köhler's disease is an osteochondrosis of the tarsal navicular bone and may present as a limp. Osteochondroses are a group of disorders that affect the growing skeleton at the ossification centres.

74   None of these statements is true

DMD is the commonest of the muscular dystrophies and is inherited in X-linked recessive fashion. The term 'muscular dystrophy' refers to a group of muscle disorders that are degenerative and inevitably progressive. The genetic defect in DMD affects the production of dystrophin, a protein that forms part of the cytoskeleton of muscle cells. DMD occurs *almost* exclusively in males, as it can occur in females with Turner's syndrome (XO) where the protective effect of the second X chromosome is missing, allowing expression of the recessive allele on the affected sex chromosome (Ferrier, *et al.*, 1965). The young child is usually slow to walk and has a tendency to fall often. Gower's sign describes the child getting up in a particular way, climbing up his or her legs because of weakness. However, this is not specific to DMD and can occur in any cause of muscle weakness. Most children will be in a wheelchair by their twelfth birthday because of the devastating progression of the illness. Up to a third of children may have concomitant learning difficulties, which may be accounted for by the presence of dystrophin in neuronal cells also. CPK levels are hugely elevated early in disease. As the disease progresses and normal muscle is replaced by redundant tissue, the CPK levels will gradually drop and may not be too far off normal. Electromyography may be useful but diagnosis is by muscle biopsy. Management revolves around maintaining independence for as long as is possible and meeting the child's social and psychological needs. Cardiorespiratory complications increase with time, and death usually occurs by the second decade of life.

75   d

Unlike JIA, a clear infective trigger is implicated in the development of acute rheumatic fever: the Lancefield group A β-haemolytic streptococcus. Diagnosis of acute rheumatic fever requires evidence of streptococcal infection (e.g. positive throat swab, history of scarlet fever, increased antistreptolysin O titre) along with either two major or one major and two minor manifestations of the Jones criteria. Chronic cardiac disease is a serious complication of rheumatic fever and the child may present with endocarditis, myocarditis or pericarditis in acute disease. A murmur on auscultation, tachycardia, bradycardia (due to partial heart block) and a pericardial friction rub all suggest cardiac involvement. In most severe cases the child may present with signs and symptoms of congestive cardiac failure. Polyarthritis may present as acutely swollen and inflamed joints or as vague joint aches and is characteristically flitting (moving around quickly) and fleeting (coming and going quickly). Larger joints are more commonly affected than smaller joints. Sydenham's chorea (also known as St Vitus's dance) is a particularly troublesome clinical manifestation of rheumatic fever. It is well recognised that there are physical and psychological aspects to the involuntary movements, which are non-repetitive, irregular and may be focal or generalised. Emotional stress may make the movements worse and they tend to disappear once the child is asleep. Overall, the chorea may have a devastating impact on the child's functional capabilities. Firm, painless subcutaneous nodules are an uncommon clinical manifestation of rheumatic fever, affecting approximately one in ten patients. They are usually involved with severe cardiac involvement. The rash associated with acute rheumatic fever is erythema marginatum. Occurring mostly on the limbs and trunk, it consists of erythematous rings with pale centres and varies in shape and site from hour to hour. Erythema multiforme consists of target lesions (red centre with surrounding pale area) and is commonly caused by infection or as a reaction to a drug.

Index

CPD with Radcliffe

You can now use a selection of our books to achieve CPD (Continuing Professional Development) points through directed reading.

We provide a free online form and downloadable certificate for your appraisal portfolio. Look for the CPD logo and register with us at: www.radcliffehealth.com/cpd

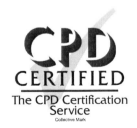

CPD CERTIFIED
The CPD Certification
Service
Collective Mark